The Meal Wheel Method for Weight Management

What Life Wants You To Know About Getting Off The Merry-Go-Round

Robin Gayle, MBA, RD, LDN, CDCES

eBook ISBN: 979-8-89420-098-9
Paperback ISBN: 979-8-89420-097-2

Library of Congress Control Number: 2026909352

CONTENTS

AUTHORS NOTE

The information in this manual is an adjunct to, not a substitute for, conventional medical therapy. It is not intended to diagnose, cure or prevent disease. The Meal Wheel Method for Weight loss is for educational purposes only and its content is not meant, in any way, as a substitute for the medical advice provided by your doctors. I strongly recommended that you always seek the advice of your physician or other qualified healthcare provider with questions regarding a medical condition or treatment before starting any weight loss program. I encourage you to share this manual with your healthcare providers prior to beginning.

Causes for overweight and obesity include genetics, environment, lifestyle choices, comorbid health conditions, stress, poor sleep and emotional factors. Nutrition is not an exact science. It should be noted that calorie intake, metabolism and level of exercise and physical exertion can vary widely from person to person. This means that weight loss results will also vary for each individual. No treatment program is effective for everyone and some individuals may not lose weight or may gain weight despite making lifestyle changes.

ACKNOWLEDGMENTS

I would like to express my eternal gratitude to the individuals who dedicated their time, energy, creativity and expertise to my project. Without them, this book would not have come to fruition. Acknowledgments are in the order that each person divinely entered this process.

To my family who gave me the tools to go out into the world and make anything happen.

To my boyfriend, Chris. Thank you for the support you have given me over the years. With you, I have the courage to go after my dreams.

To Jane Nester, beloved friend. Thank you for reading through the early stages of my manuscript before any formal editing was done. That could not have been easy. All jokes aside, your feedback, suggestions, and support for my endeavor were greatly appreciated. You have been a wonderful mentor to me both in my career as well as my life. I feel truly blessed to have you on my life journey.

To Beth Carmichael, the first editor to review my manuscript. Many thanks for agreeing to get the ball rolling. I learned so much about the editing process from you. Your feedback and guidance were presented with such kindness. That quality was so important to me as a vulnerable new author. Thank you from the bottom of my heart.

To Jimmy Hamill, the second editor to review my manuscript. Heartfelt thanks for agreeing to pick up the editing where Beth left off. I will always remember and appreciate your willingness to jump in and help.

To Dr. Joel Rosenfeld, dear friend and esteemed colleague. Special thanks for your sincere interest in my project. The hours of line editing that you provided were invaluable and greatly appreciated. I admire your dedication to seeing it through to the end. Thank you for believing in me.

To Tara Furniss, my dear friend. Thank you for taking the time to read my manuscript and provide a genuine critique of the material from the perspective of my demographic. Your enthusiasm and belief in me mean the world to me. I feel especially lucky to have shared this experience with you.

To Jona Kottler, editor, and new friend, I will be forever indebted to you for bringing my manuscript together to create a cohesive book. Your creativity and expertise are exceptional. I learned so much from working with you and thoroughly enjoyed the process. It was not a coincidence that I found you. You are truly the best.

To my publishers, for taking my book to publication.

The Meal Wheel Method for Weight Management

PREFACE

There are about as many weight-loss plans out there as there are messages about how you need to lose weight to get your body ready for summer, to make a New Year's resolution to really do it this time, or fit yourself into a Hollywood ideal. We are bombarded every day with ways to "melt belly fat" and "speed up our metabolism effortlessly after forty."

No one can motivate you to make real, long-term changes in your weight but yourself. I'll bet that since you picked up this book today, you are already familiar with lots of different ways you've been told will "fix" you. Some of them want to simplify foods into small units so that you don't have to worry about what you're eating. Some of them want you to eliminate whole groups of foods entirely. Some only want to let you eat at certain times of day, or portion your meals into little packets. All of these take away stress about food so you don't have to think.

I want to **give** you something instead of taking anything away. I want to give you the knowledge you need to make active, informed choices about what you eat. I want to give you insight not just about food, but about your relationship with food, and ways to heal that relationship that will help you to make great choices to fuel your body and be happier. Not just because you'll lose weight (you **will lose weight!**) but because you're the one controlling how you feel about food instead of having food control you.

The Meal Wheel Method puts the power in your hands and focuses on the connection between your mind and your body. Instead of taking things away, or oversimplifying important concepts, being informed about how your body uses food to fuel itself, and how your mind and emotions can help you rather than hinder you puts you firmly in the driver's seat of your own health.

As a licensed and registered dietitian, I have worked with thousands of patients over the years and have had many people return to my office just to tell me their success stories, which include weight losses of up to eighty pounds, increased energy levels to do their daily activities, boosts in self-confidence, and an overall improvement in their sense of wellbeing. They are often amazed at their own resilience to overcome difficulty which provides them with an added level of pride and self-respect. What I have come to realize through my patient experiences is that most people simply don't understand the basics of healthy eating. I started thinking about the useful information I could share with others. Information that can help everyone understand the fundamentals of food the way a dietitian does. In turn, I can help people maintain a healthier weight.

On many occasions I've heard, "I thought this visit was going to be a lot worse. What you just showed me doesn't seem that hard. No one has ever explained it to me that way before. I really think I can do this." Of course, hearing that makes me very happy! It also makes me realize that I could never meet with as many people individually as I would like, but I could create the next best thing—the Meal Wheel and book—to guide people through the process, just as if I were seeing them as patients. The Meal Wheel is a simple tool that will help you understand how much food from each food group to consume at meals and snacks. It's a straightforward way of controlling calories without necessarily counting calories. I like to think I am providing a target for you to aim at after shooting in the dark for so long. You don't have to hit the bullseye. You just have to get close to the target to see results. Couple the Meal Wheel with this book, and you will understand precisely what you need to work on and what it takes to create a healthy balanced diet.

Most people want to improve their health and/or appearance in some way. Through my work over the years, I have met numerous individuals who have expressed that desire. My observation has been that once you know how to use the Meal Wheel to eat properly, the other barriers to losing weight fall somewhere between ***wanting*** the weight loss and ***doing*** what it takes to achieve the change in weight. We get stuck between wanting and doing. If you think about *resistance* and look for the path of least resistance for you to obtain what you want, you'll find the answer to your success—even though it might not be the easiest solution. In a perfect world, for example, the path of least resistance would be to stop all the dietary indiscretions that cause some weight problems (snacking on goodies and eating fast food, etc.) and always make the "right" choice. We all realize, however, that humans are not perfect and we do not live in a perfect world. The good news is that if you find your path somewhere between what I suggest and your present habits, you will start to experience positive change. Following the Meal Wheel recommendations, even partially, allows you to start your journey while still enjoying an occasional treat. In fact, if you allow yourself to have snacks occasionally, you will establish a more reasonable relationship with food as opposed to telling yourself that you can never have "goodies" again, which may lead to feelings of deprivation and the desire to consume them even more.

My role as a dietitian is to assist my patients' understanding of how food affects their bodies. The patients themselves must learn how to navigate all the emotions that accompany a weight loss program. It is natural to react and feel uncomfortable when change appears to threaten our status quo. It is something we all have experienced, and I have seen it many times with my patients. The difference between those individuals who are successful and those who don't quite reach their goal is how well they negotiate conflict resolution, how much they want a positive outcome, and how much they want to continue their usual habits. Investigating the feelings that are brought to the surface during this process and creating more awareness of them is something I will discuss more in the "Food for Thought" section of the book. This book is a blend of practical advice, philosophy, counseling, and encouragement. My goal is to help you be successful. To do this you will need to do two things: (1) use the Meal Wheel and this hands-on book about what and how much to eat, and (2) tap into your will and mental strength to stick with the plan — which will become easier when you start listening to your thoughts and start changing them.

WHAT TO EXPECT:

1. The nuts and bolts of your body's nutritional needs and how the Meal Wheel System will make it so that making good choices comes easily.
2. A step-by-step method for finding the perfect personalized formula for supporting your body while you meet your goals for healthy weight loss.
3. Exercises to help you understand your emotional relationship with food and ways to improve that relationship.
4. The Meal Wheel itself is a simple, powerful tool that puts control over your choices right into your own hands.
5. All about Janet[1]: the story of one of my patients from the first day she decided to change her relationship with food--you will find lots of common challenges and triumphs that your own story shares with hers.
6. My own story--overcoming a difficult relationship with

[1] "Janet" is a composite character based on my experience with patients.

food shares so many traits with overcoming anxiety, which was a challenge I had to face.

No matter why you have decided that you want to take the journey to better health, there are tools in this book to support and empower you. I'm excited to guide you and help you to make your life the way you want it to be.

So, let's go!

CHAPTER ONE: WHY TODAY?

There's something special about today. Someone made an offhand comment about how you look in those pants. You saw a photo of yourself from Thanksgiving that someone posted on social media. Perhaps you've heard from a doctor that you have to lose ten percent of your body weight before you can have the surgery that you need. Whether you're motivated by the way you look or the way you feel, today is the day that you've decided to make a change. Maybe you've even tried before, and felt like a failure, either because you couldn't make sense of a weight loss plan, or because you lost some weight and then gained it all back (or all of it plus a few more). Today the Meal Wheel system is going to help you to change your life.

But let's be realistic. The Meal Wheel system is fantastic (if I do say so myself, and I do because I've developed it and used it to help thousands of patients) but it's not magic. It's a framework for changing your life, and the key part of that word is **work**.

First, let's tackle some questions you might want to ask yourself. I recommend starting a special file on your computer or phone or buying a journal that you really like, as a place to record the answers to questions, journal about how you're feeling, make notes about meals that made you happy, or ways you're feeling frustrated on your journey.

Start by answering these questions:

- Why today? What has brought you to the decision that you are ready to put in the effort to lose weight?
- What do you imagine you will feel like when you reach your goal?
- What are the things that you are afraid of in starting this journey?
- What has held you back every day before today?
- Write a list of words that come to your mind when you think about losing weight.
- How was food regarded in your family of origin? Was it a way of showing love? A bribe? A punishment?
- What are the ways that your family of origin's food values impacted you then? Impact you now?
- What are your favorite foods? When do you eat them? Why do you eat them?
- What talents and strengths do you have in other areas of your life that you think you can apply to your health journey?
- What's your relationship to exercise? When did it start?
- In what ways do you enjoy moving your body?

Answering these questions will help you to assess your beliefs. By taking a good, hard look at yourself you will be able to notice some of the key beliefs that often stop people from making positive, long-term changes to their diet. They will help you to apply the practical steps of the Meal Wheel program more successfully to your daily life, and help you understand better how you can take control of your relationship with food and movement.

In order to be successful in the weight loss process, you must be open to giving up your old beliefs and habits. Most of them have not worked for you in the past (that's why you are here looking for something new!) and they are not likely to work for you in the future. Weight loss is a mind game. If you can't change your mind, you can't change your weight. To quote Irish playwright and Nobel prize winner in literature George Bernard Shaw, "Those who cannot change their minds cannot change anything."[2] Working on governing your thoughts will prove beneficial and make this journey easier and much more rewarding than you can imagine. In the end, only you have the power to change your thought process and achieve your goals.

The most important point I would like you to understand is that *you have complete control over your weight loss quest*. You make all the decisions here, not the family that you came from, not your friends, not even your past self. When faced with a difficult decision, there are only two paths: what you choose to do and what you choose not to do. I'm here to help you feel

---

[2] George Bernard Shaw, *Everybody's Political What's What*, (London: Constable and Company Ltd., 1944), 330.

empowered, with facts, pro tips, and stories for those times when you feel like you can't do it because your mind has you believing the situation is out of your control. When you are completely honest with yourself, you will find that you can do almost anything you set your mind to. The thoughts you have about your weight or weight loss or your past or your future are keeping you trapped right where you are at present.

Here is your first opportunity to dip your toes in the pool of possibilities. Examine your beliefs. Put them under a microscope. I encourage you to ponder your present assumptions on weight loss. Begin to re-evaluate them. Our beliefs about everything are shaped by our own ideas and perceptions as well as influenced by what we see. This is certainly true about what we see and hear about food and weight loss. Some common and, unfortunately, very restrictive beliefs I have heard over the years include the following:

1. Eating healthy is too hard.
2. Eating healthy is too expensive.
3. I love food too much.
4. I've tried to lose weight before and nothing works.
5. I feel like I'm being punished.
6. Other people get to eat whatever they want, and they don't have weight problems.
7. I don't have time to exercise.
8. What's the use, I will probably regain the weight anyway.

The good news is that you can re-work this negative thinking into something affirmative and create a forward motion in your life. According to Joe Dispenza, neuroscientist and author of "Breaking the Habit of Being Yourself: How to Lose Your Mind and Create a New One":

> "Our routine, known thoughts, and feelings perpetuate the same state of being, which creates the same behaviors and creates the same reality. If we want to change some aspect of our reality, we have to think, feel, and act in new ways; we have to "be" different in terms of our responses to experiences. We have to create a new state of mind and observe a new outcome with that new mind."[3]

Simply put, we need to reprogram our thought patterns, as well as our actions, into ones that are more aligned with what we want and how we will get it.

Before we get into the details of using the Meal Wheel to portion out our foods and create meal plans, let's analyze some of the beliefs listed above that may run through our minds, as this type of thinking can greatly influence our accomplishments as well as our failures. A considerable problem with thoughts is that we confuse them with facts. I would like you to challenge your

---

[3] Dr. Joe Dispenza, Breaking the Habit of Being Yourself: How to Lose Your Mind and Create a New One, (Carlsbad, CA: Hay House, Inc., 2012), 22.

thoughts, rather than allow them to direct you. When I do this in my own life, I'm always surprised by what I learn.

I will start with the belief that eating healthy is too expensive – a statement that I frequently hear. Recent research, however, is finding that eating healthy may not be as expensive as one might think. According to the USDA, the price of food is calculated in three ways: the price per calorie, per edible gram, and per average portion. It is also dependent on the specific foods being compared. Per the USDA, "regardless of the metric used, the analysis makes clear that it is not possible to conclude that healthy foods are more expensive than less healthy food[4]."

Using a straightforward real-life example and taking a closer look in practical terms, we will find that eating junk food can be equally, if not more, expensive. Let's put our money where our mouth is and dare to compare what twenty dollars can buy! While it is outside the scope of this book (which is not a cookbook), there are many resources available that address how to shop and meal plan on a budget and how to prepare dishes that are Meal Wheel compatible. Once you are used to eating according to the Meal Wheel plan, you'll be able to adapt these

---

[4] Andrea Carlson and Elizabeth Frazão, *Are Healthy Foods Really More Expensive? It depends on How You Measure the Price*, EIB-96, U.S. Department of Agriculture, Economic Research Service, May 2012, 30.

tips and recipes to your own needs. Remember to look for books and sites that provide whole food recipes and guidelines, not fad diets.

McDonald's® (meal for two people)[5]

Two double quarter pounders with cheese	$6.39 x 2 = $12.78	1480 calories
Two medium chocolate milkshakes	$3.99 x 2 = $7.98	1260 calories
Two large French fries	$3.25 x 2 = $6.50	1600 calories
Three chocolate chip cookies	$1.25	510 calories
Total	**$28.51**	**4850 calories**

Food Store

One loaf of 100% Whole Wheat Bread	$5.29	440 calories/ 4 slices
Three cans of Chunk Light Tuna in water	$4.47	300 calories/ 1 can
A three-pound bag of Gala apples	$4.99	160 calories/ 2 apples
11.5 oz light mayonnaise	$4.99	35 calories/ 1 Tbsp
Total	**$19.74**	**935 calories**/ 2 sandwiches made

---

[5] McDonalds. Menu. N.d. https://www.mcdonalds.com/us/en-us/full-menu/burgers.html

		with one can of tuna and two apples

Looking at this comparison, we find that we get substantially more value with the healthy food store choices, as two people could each consume tuna fish sandwiches and apples for three days and still have bread and apples leftover to use for more lunches. Not only is the healthy choice more cost-effective, but it contains less than one-quarter the calories of the fast-food lunch! You may have to trade off convenience for a little bit of effort, but it will be worth it in the end.

There are also hidden costs to unhealthy eating. We just don't always connect the cost of medicine, doctor's appointments, or not feeling well with our comparison of the cost of food. Did you know that people with a diagnosis of obesity, which is defined as a Body Mass Index (BMI) of $\geq$ 30, spend an additional $1723 annually on medical expenses associated with obesity? The direct medical cost of being overweight, with a BMI of 24.9-29.9, is an extra $266 of medical spending a year. While being overweight is correlated with a more modest expense, it may only be so in the short term and may very well increase with time[6].

---

[6] Abhilasha Ramasamy et al., "Direct and Indirect Cost of Obesity Among the Privately Insured in the United States." *Journal of Occupational and Environmental Medicine* 61, no. 11 (November 2019): 877-886. doi: 10.1097/JOM.0000000000001693.

Another common belief many people have is that they don't have enough time to work out. I have certainly been guilty of this way of thinking. What I have come to realize is that there is usually time in my week to exercise. I advise my patients to keep a time log and record how they spend their time during the day. I strongly suggest that you do this too. Begin from the time you wake up till you go to sleep, seven days a week. This type of time tracker is very similar to a food tracker. It will demonstrate where you are not being efficient with your time. Where are you engaging in mindless activity? What activities can you cut back on that are not enhancing your life (i.e., watching television, shopping online, or using social media apps) to create more time to be productive? How could you use the habits that you already have (like watching tv) to help you rather than hurt you? What about saving a favorite show to watch only on the treadmill? Lifting weights during commercials? Start ranking exercise higher on your list of things to do and watch how much you accomplish.

I would like to point out that *not having time* to exercise and *not feeling like* exercising are two different dilemmas. We have to be willing to differentiate between the two. If you find that you don't feel like exercising, it may be because you are not used to doing it and it's easier and more convenient to keep doing what you are accustomed to doing. This conclusion is fine if there are no expectations of improving your health or your body. The reality is if you keep doing what you are doing you will keep getting the same result, so it's time to change how you think about it.

Finally, I'd like to address the importance of re-examining your beliefs and why this critical work is a part of using the Meal Wheel. And yes, I mean it when I say that it is work. Let's consider the perception that "other people get to eat whatever they want, and they don't have a weight problem." I am sure some people stay thin no matter what they consume. I do not believe that this is the norm. Most people need to put in some effort to maintain a normal weight especially as they get older. Just because a person seems to be able to eat whatever type of food that they want without it having an impact on their weight does not mean that their body is healthy. It is possible that when a person gains weight, their body is communicating to them that they need to address an issue with their nutrition as well as their belief system. A thin person does not get a warning sign and may not be aware that they need to change their eating habits.

The bottom line is none of us know for certain what another person goes through in their life. We don't know their eating or exercise habits, and we don't know their medical history or genetic background. To compare your circumstances to another person's life is a recipe for misery. It implies that someone else is the "lucky or special one," and that you are the unfortunate one, the victim of your circumstances, doomed to remain overweight. Essentially, this way of thinking is a way of absolving yourself of any responsibility regarding the choices you make, since you believe the choice has already been made for you. If you allow any of the above thoughts to dominate your thinking, your overweight situation will persist. If you change the dialogue and visualize working on a healthier and more fit body, that is what you will obtain. We always get what we predominantly think about.

Food can't hold you back; it's just food. There is no power in food. But your thoughts about food can definitely limit you. Thinking you "love" food holds you back--you can enjoy food! Why wouldn't you? It's delicious and it's one of the pleasures of life. But thinking that food is worthy of the same emotion that we reserve for the people in our lives isn't going to help you adjust your relationship to it. Thinking that you'll be happy if you look a certain way holds you back. We will delve back into the important ways that our feelings can sabotage our weight management further in the book, but for the present, it is critical to understand that you have given food power that it just doesn't possess. Of course, we need food for the purpose it was meant to have—to nourish the body. It is not intended to control our lives. Only you can change that old worn-out recording. You may not even be conscious of the recording. Start to develop awareness around your thoughts and habits and see all the wonderful opportunities that arise from them. Each moment provides the chance to think a different way!

TODAY IS THE DAY FOR JANET

Janet is fifty-one years old. When she was younger, she

used to describe herself as "plump" or "fluffy." She put on the regulation freshman fifteen when she went to college, and she has raised two children, each of which left her with some extra pounds after her pregnancies. She wasn't thrilled to be heavier, but she was amazed at the strength and power of her own body, bringing her boys into the world and nurturing them. Now with the boys settled into their own adult lives, she is busy with her job, friends, and hobbies. She'd never wear a bikini, but her husband loves her and she is content with her life.

Last week, Janet woke up with pain in her neck and jaw. She's guilty of doing what we all do; she did an online search of her symptoms and began to worry that she wasn't just stressed out because of the big project that she was on deadline for at work but that she was actually having early symptoms of a heart attack. Janet's father had a heart attack when he was fifty; a year younger than she is. Thinking about all of this made her scared, and she started to feel a heaviness in her chest that could have been anxiety--or something worse.

Janet made the trip to Urgent Care where she had an EKG and blood test. She found out that her heart looked good and that there were no markers in her blood that showed she'd had a heart attack. Of course, she was relieved, but she was also motivated. Clipping off the white hospital band from her wrist, Janet took the Urgent Care doctor's advice and contacted me. Today was the day that she decided she would make a change.

When I meet with a new patient, I always start with one question: "What are you hoping to gain from this visit?" It is a very important question that some people have given thought to prior to their visit, while others haven't given it any consideration. A common answer is, "My doctor wanted me to meet with the dietitian." I want you to think about what it is you want to achieve and why it is important to you. Make a list of your answers to the question "why"—why is managing my weight significant to me? When the road gets rough and you feel like you are losing momentum, you can revisit your list to remind yourself of the value of accomplishing your goals. Your list will provide you with the strength to press on. Common themes on many of my patients' lists include reasons like:

I want to be healthier.

I want to ensure my quality of life as I age.

I want to feel better about myself.

I want to live to see my children graduate, get married, etc.

I want to be able to play with my grandchildren.

What does your list look like?

It's worth making this list because you are the most important person in your life. Now is the time to make an investment in defining and accomplishing your goals, because you are the one who counts here. You are the only one that can make change happen and get things done. Here are some rules that are meant to help keep you realistic and optimistic:

SIMPLE RULES OF THE MEAL WHEEL: THE BAKER'S DOZEN

1. The Meal Wheel is not a magic wheel. For the best results, follow the instructions to the best of your ability.
2. Take time to develop your meal plans ahead of mealtime based on the Meal Wheel recommendations. This is a process that requires dedicated learning time each day to review your plan for the day, ensuring that you have everything you need to be successful for that day.
3. Blow the dust off your measuring cups and measuring spoons. Use them. They are not the enemy. I keep my measuring cups alongside the sink where they are visible, convenient, and can easily be rinsed off after I use them.
4. Accept the fact that you may occasionally feel a little hungry. This is a normal sensation associated with consuming less food. Nothing bad will happen by responsibly decreasing your calorie intake. You can use the Portion Guide, found on page 201-212 of the book, for the list of free foods to consume to help you feel full.
5. Please consume three meals a day. If you don't want to, this may not be the program for you. Balancing your food intake throughout the day is critical to successful weight loss and long-term weight management.

6. Record, record, record! Keep track of your daily intake. There are plenty of apps, such as MyFitnessPal, that you can use to make it easy to track your intake. It is vital to know what you are consuming and there is really no way to understand what you are doing unless you keep a daily food diary.
7. Closely examine your thoughts and your present habits. I have learned that it is not as much about the food we eat as it is about the thoughts and habits that drive us to consume the food. Learn to think about food in the same way you think about filling up the tank of your car. It is time to refuel. Eating is something you do to give yourself energy when your body's tank is low. It is just that simple!
8. Listen to yourself. If after the first week of using your Meal Wheel, you find yourself saying, "This doesn't work," tell yourself to *STOP*. That is your self-sabotaging mind doing what it does best. You will not see results from this program in one week. This is an endurance test. You win the race by staying the course.
9. Don't compare yourself to others. That is a true prescription for unhappiness. This is your individual journey, and no one else matters in this situation. Elements that affect the rate of weight loss include our gender and genetic background, amount of lean muscle mass, present metabolic state, medications we may be taking, and physical limitations to exercise.

10. Accept that losing one pound a week is GREAT! In one year, that equates to fifty-two pounds! You may think that is a long time, but consider how long it took you to gain that weight.
11. Move your body every day. Exercise is an integral part of weight management. It makes you feel good! Did you know that according to the National Weight Control Registry (NWCR), exercise is the number one indicator for successful weight loss maintenance?[7]
12. I have good news for you! Whether you believe it or not, you are perfect just as you are in this present moment. Remind yourself daily of all the wonderful things that are working for you in your life and acknowledge that every day you are getting healthier and healthier.
13. Finally, always be kind to yourself. You owe it to yourself. Now, let's get to work!

THE NUTRITION CONSULT

When an individual comes to see me for a one-on-one consultation, we begin by discussing what brings the client to me. During this initial hour-long visit, I like to take my time getting to

---

[7] Rena R. Wing and Suzanne Phelan, "Long-term weight loss maintenance." *The American Journal of Clinical Nutrition* 82, no. 1 (2005): 222S-225S. https://doi.org/10.1093/ajcn/82.1.222S.

know the patient's experience with dieting and how they feel about making lifestyle changes. Then, I address the following topics:

1. The food recall
2. Calculating body weight
3. Calculating calorie needs
4. The food groups
5. Goal setting

The food recall tends to be the bulk of the first visit. This is how I learn the individual's food habits. I calculate body weight and calorie needs on my own prior to the visit, teach you the information that you will need, and show you how to use it a bit later in the book.

THE FOOD RECALL

The food recall provides me with an idea of what a patient's present eating habits are. It helps me with approximating how many calories they are consuming on a daily basis. I use the food recall as a baseline, or a starting point, to identify problem areas and determine where we can start making changes. The food recall is my way of initiating the awareness process around the individual's food practices. It usually uncovers where excess calories and other dietary problems exist.

Since I am not there with you in person, you'll need to do your own food recall by writing down everything you normally eat and drink in a day – a food log. I recommend that you do this for several days prior to making any changes to get a better picture of what you are ***actually eating***, rather than what you ***think*** you are eating. Be sure to include the amounts of ***everything*** you have consumed, as you will go back to your food recall later and compare it to the meal plan you choose from your Meal Wheel. This will help you to differentiate what you are doing and what the Meal Wheel is recommending. This comparison is a real eye-opener. It will help you decide where you can start making meaningful dietary modifications. For now, complete your three-day food log as shown in the example below. A blank food log is provided in Appendix D at the back of the book. You can make copies of it to track your food intake. Of course, you may use any tracking system you like as long as you initiate the process.

SAMPLE FOOD RECALL:

TIME	**FOOD**	**AMOUNT CONSUMED**
9:30 a.m.	Eggs, scrambled in butter	2 2 tsp
	Scrapple	3 oz.
	Home fries	1 cup
	Rye bread toasted	2 slices
	Butter	1 Tbsp.
	Tomato juice	8 oz.

	Coffee	12 oz.
	Creamer	2 Tbsp
	Artificial sweetener	1 packet
12:30 p.m.	Mixed greens	2 cups
	Grilled chicken breast	4 oz.
	Caesar salad dressing	¼ cup
	Diet soda	12 oz.
7:30 p.m.	Wheat pasta, cooked	2 cups
	Marinara sauce	¾ cup
	Meatballs, brand x	4 oz.
	Salad	1 cup
	Ranch dressing	¼ cup
	Diet soda	12 oz.
8:30 p.m.	Ice cream	1 cup

Now that you have a fairly accurate and detailed account of what you normally eat, it's time to take a closer look at your current dietary habits. It's important to have a critical eye when evaluating your food record to identify the main areas you need to address. When I review a food record, I am generally looking for two main points: is the person consuming regular meals at regular times, and are the meals balanced? Other common habits that I want you to watch for include inconsistent carbohydrate intake at meals, large portion sizes, excess calories coming from fat, and the frequency of meals consumed outside of the house and/or consumption of take-out/fast food. Let's practice!

How would you evaluate this sample food recall above? My brief scan of this food log reveals poorly timed meals, inconsistent carbohydrate intake, lack of balanced meals, and excess calories coming from high-fat food choices. Let's review each of these problems and discuss them one-by-one.

1. Consuming three meals a day cannot be stressed enough. Our bodies work most efficiently when we fuel them at regular intervals throughout the day. An individual would, preferably, consume three meals a day about four to five hours apart. This individual allowed seven hours to pass between lunch and dinner creating the potential to overeat at the next meal due to hunger. Skipping meals will create a similar situation. When we feel hungry, we are more likely to snack and overeat. Therefore, consuming regular meals at regular times will not only help control hunger, but it will also control calorie intake.
2. Inconsistent carbohydrate intake means that this individual included carbohydrates at breakfast and dinner, but they did not have any carbohydrates at lunch. Further, they had approximately sixty grams of carbohydrates at breakfast and over one hundred grams at dinner (this person likely over-ate due to inadequate intake at lunch). Ideally, this person would be fueling his/her body with about the same amount of

carbohydrates at each meal to control calorie intake, aid with satiety, and promote an optimally functioning metabolism.

3. This person's intake lacks balanced meals. People are better able to meet their nutrient needs if they consume balanced meals that include some carbohydrates, protein, and fat. They will feel more satiated, helping them get from one meal to the next without feeling too hungry between meals. Balance is needed to ensure we are getting all the vital nutrients our body requires while being mindful of the nutrients that should be limited. Balance also signifies that we are not over-consuming a particular nutrient. Following the Meal Wheel recommendations for carbohydrates, protein, and fat will ensure that we meet our nutrient requirements while maintaining the calorie control needed to produce weight loss.
4. Excess calories from fat can thwart all efforts towards losing weight. We are so preoccupied with carbohydrates that we forget the impact of the other macronutrients. Fat has more than twice as many calories as carbohydrates and protein. Even seemingly small amounts can ruin a diet (more on this later!).

These are the items I would point out at the visit and ask the client to modify. I normally conclude the visit by reinforcing the importance of focusing on what to eat, when to eat, and how much to eat. We then set goals based on the main issues that we pinpointed.

CHAPTER TWO: FOOD AND YOU

We all know the big truth here: our relationship to food has a huge impact on how we feel about ourselves, and how food impacts our lives and our weight. We can't just quit food cold turkey (look, even our language and the way we express non-food ideas uses food words!), so in order to have successful weight loss with long-term maintenance, we have to examine the facts about food and the emotions connected to it. In the last chapter, I had you answer some questions about why you are starting this journey, how food was regarded in your family, and how you feel about movement. Now I'd like you to consider some of the ways that you feel about food itself:

- Are there such things as "good" and "bad" foods? Which foods fit into which category? What do you think about yourself when you eat "good" foods versus when you eat "bad" ones?
- How do you feel when you are eating something you really love? Does the feeling increase the more you eat that something?
- Do you eat food as a way to reward yourself for doing something difficult? What do you eat? How do you feel when you eat it? How do you feel after?
- What are the foods you associate with special occasions? How often do you have these foods? (For example, once a

year during the holiday season, once a year at birthdays, once a month, etc.)

- Do you ever feel that you have to eat something to be polite, or to not call attention to yourself/your weight? How do you feel when you eat that?
- Do you ever eat secretly? A hidden candy bar? A fast-food burger that you eat in the car and then hide the wrappers? If you do, why do you feel that you need to hide it? What would happen if someone found out? How do you feel when you are eating the food? How do you feel after?
- Do you ever eat food unconsciously? A treat from the break room? A bagel at a meeting that's gone without you remembering that you ate it? A few candies from the bowl on someone's desk? A few chips or bites left on a child's plate when you are clearing up the dishes?
- Were you told as a child that wasting food was a bad thing and that you had to clear your plate? Do you carry that with you still? Pass it on to your own kids?
- Have you ever had to eat something you didn't want to eat because you knew it would hurt someone if you didn't?

Food is neutral. It doesn't speak to your morals or your worth. It's fuel that your body uses to keep itself going. It's **people** that connect values to food; sometimes great ones like a special recipe that you make every year to celebrate, sometimes problematic ones that say that you wouldn't "look like this," "be so bad," or "have this problem" if you could "just control yourself." As you're considering all those emotional values that people attach to food and the consumption of food, I want you to have the facts about food.

THE FOOD GROUPS

I don't believe that any one food group is better or worse than another. I treat all food groups equally, as they each serve an important function in our diet. I am truly astonished when people tell me they avoid certain food groups—unless they have a medical reason. It is hard for me to even imagine not consuming a variety of foods. I often ask people to close their eyes and think about what is in the foods they avoid that they think will hurt them. Is it the vitamins and minerals? Is it the water content of the food? Is it the disease-fighting antioxidants and phytochemicals? Is it the carbohydrate content? I want to tap into their belief system to better understand their thoughts and what is required for them to begin changing their minds.

It's important to examine your opinions about food and where they originated. Why do you believe that carbohydrates are bad? What suggests to you that a diet high in protein is better? Are you afraid that eating fatty foods will make you fat? It's time to start thinking about food differently. Now is the time to commit to a more balanced intake that includes all the wonderful food groups. I sincerely believe that variety will make it easier to support a meal plan over the long term, and will make you a happier, healthier person.

CARBOHYDRATES: THE BASICS

Carbohydrates have a bad reputation in our culture (other foods have had a turn being the villains—in the 1990 fat was the baddie, which led to a whole kind of diet revolution that took fat content out of foods like cookies and brownies, and replaced it with heaps of sugar). Carbohydrates are macronutrients. Macronutrients are nutrients that add caloric value to our diet. Protein and fat are **also** considered macronutrients. Most of the calories we consume in our diet (fifty percent or more) commonly come from carbohydrates. Carbohydrates are sugar, starch, and fiber. They provide four calories per gram. One hundred percent of the carbohydrates we consume are digested and broken down into glucose. This glucose then goes into the bloodstream, where it is taken up by the body's cells and burned as fuel to provide the energy we need to live. I compare this process to putting gasoline into the tank of a car. If you don't put gas in the tank, then the car will not run. If you put bad gas in the tank, then the car will run poorly or may even be ruined. Like a car, the body needs the appropriate energy source to run properly. This energy source primarily comes from carbohydrates.

Most carbohydrates are good for us if we consume the right kinds in the right amounts. They are derived from three main food groups: starch, fruit, and low-fat dairy. Examples of wholesome carbohydrates include whole grain bread and pasta, brown rice, quinoa, fresh fruit as well as no-sugar-added frozen fruit, and low-fat milk and yogurt.

The carbs that aren't in the "best kind" category, like sweets and fried foods such as French fries and chips often constitute a significant part of many people's daily intake. They are nutrient-poor and full of "empty" calories, which are primary culprits in the struggle with our weight. Empty carbohydrates that ***are not*** nourishing to our overall health include many packaged, processed, and fast foods as well as items made from white flour, including white breads and pasta. Foods that contain refined sugar, such as candy, cakes, cookies, pies, ice cream, and sugar-sweetened beverages, need to be strictly limited, if not avoided altogether, to maintain a healthy weight.[8]

PROTEIN: THE BASICS

People often think that protein is a "free" food that has the magical power of immediate weight loss. While protein doesn't possess superpowers, it is an important nutrient as it is part of every cell in the body and is used to build and repair all body tissues. Protein breaks down into smaller components called amino acids and contains four calories per gram. Many of the amino acids that make up protein are synthesized by the body. The

---

[8] Joanne L. Slavin and Justin Carlson, "Carbohydrates." *Advances in Nutrition* 5, no. 6 (Nov. 2014): 760-1. doi: 10.3945/an.114.006163.

ones that are not manufactured by the body are considered essential amino acids and must be obtained through the foods we eat.

Dietary sources of protein can either be plant-based or animal-based protein. Animal-based proteins are considered complete proteins because they contain all of the essential amino acids. They are found in all animal tissue such as chicken, beef, or fish, as well as anything derived from an animal such as eggs, milk, yogurt, and cheese. Plant-based proteins, on the other hand, are considered incomplete because they are missing one or more of the essential amino acids. The good news is that you can create a complete protein by combining complementary proteins found in a variety of beans and grains. Examples of complementary proteins include rice and beans or peanut butter on whole-grain toast. What's more, you don't have to consume the complementary proteins in the same meal. You can consume the beans on your salad at lunch and rice with dinner and your body can still combine them to create a complete protein!

Focus on choosing lean proteins such as poultry, fish, and low-fat meats and cheeses. You can even toss in a vegetarian meal or two during the week and meet your protein needs.[9]

---

[9] National Research Council (US) Subcommittee on the Tenth Edition of the Recommended Dietary Allowances, "Protein and Amino Acids" in

FAT: THE BASICS

Fat is an essential nutrient that our bodies require for normal function. As I mentioned earlier, when a nutrient is "essential," it means that we need to consume it through the food we eat because our bodies cannot synthesize it on their own. Fat provides us with the essential fatty acids that our bodies depend upon. The problem here is that we consume **far more** fat in the form of both added fat and naturally occurring fat than we require. The extra calories from fat make it harder to maintain a healthy weight.

Fat is also the most calorically dense of the macronutrients, providing nine calories per gram. Both carbohydrates and protein provide only four calories per gram. A smaller amount of fat, therefore, quickly adds up to more calories. I find that fat calories often sneak into our diet without us realizing it. Nuts are a great example of this. A serving of cashews, for instance, is six nuts. Yes, six nuts! I have had clients who snack on a cup of nuts in front of the TV every night, and they don't realize there are roughly eight hundred calories in that cup of nuts they are eating. If they were to cut back to a one-half cup serving, they could theoretically lose three-quarters of a pound a week just by

---

Recommended Dietary Allowances, 10th Edition. (Washington, DC: National Academies Press, 1989), 52-77.

consuming the smaller portion! They could lose one and a half pounds a week if they eliminate that snack altogether.

Also, be sure to choose lean meats and low-fat cheese, as we tend to get a significant amount of fat in our diet from animal protein. Paying attention to your added fat choices at each meal and staying within the Meal Wheel parameters will work wonders with calorie control.[10]

PROCESSED FOODS

Processed foods are important because we rely on them mainly for their convenience. They are foods that have been altered in some way from their original form. The word "processed" is often thought to have negative connotations, but this is not always true. In fact, there are plenty of processed foods that maintain their integrity while being made more convenient for us to use. Processed can refer to foods that have been cut, mashed, juiced, frozen, canned, cooked, preserved, or otherwise manipulated. We process food daily when we prepare and cook a meal. If you mashed potatoes and tenderized your meat, you processed food. I opt for freshly cut and packaged pineapple at my grocery store. These manipulations are perfectly reasonable ways

---

[10] "Healthy Diet," World Health Organization, Apr. 29, 2020, https://www.who.int/news-room/fact-sheets/detail/healthy-diet.

to prepare your food.

The problem is that not all processed foods are created equal. For instance, there is a significant difference between the dinner you put together at home and the frozen meal you purchase at the grocery store. Processed food can fall anywhere on a scale from minimally processed to ultra-processed. Let's take a look at examples of foods that fall into the different categories.

NOVA is a food classification system that categorizes food based on how it is processed. It was created by the Center for Epidemiological Studies in Health and Nutrition at the School of Public Health, University of Sao Paulo, Brazil. According to their own description of the institution, "NOVA helps people group foods according to the extent and purpose of the processing they undergo." Food processing identified by NOVA involves physical, biological, and chemical processes that occur after foods are separated from nature and before they are consumed or used in the preparation of dishes and meals. The system identifies the following four levels of food manipulation:

1. **Unprocessed or minimally processed foods** are picked and consumed without any change. An orange off a tree, a head of lettuce from the garden, or raspberries off the bush are all examples of unprocessed foods. Minimally processed is when fruits or vegetables are picked and put into a bag to be sold in a store. Fresh green beans or baby carrots in a bag are minimally processed foods.

2. Processed culinary ingredients are obtained from unprocessed foods and are altered through processes such as pressing or grinding to be used for cooking. Pressing olives to make olive oil is an example of a processed culinary ingredient.

3. Lightly processed foods are, for example, fruits and vegetables that are canned or frozen shortly after being picked. They often contain two or three added ingredients, such as salt or sugar. Other examples include breads, cheeses, and pasta.

4. Ultra-processed foods are made with five or more ingredients, such as salt, fat, sugar, stabilizers, and preservatives. Examples of ultra-processed foods are frozen meals, pizza, snack foods such as chips, cookies, and cakes, sugar-sweetened cereals, and soft drinks. All foods in this category are considered unhealthy. They are associated with an increased risk for obesity, diabetes, and cardiovascular disease. I recommend that you avoid foods in this category.[11]

Try and choose unprocessed or minimally processed foods at the store. You can do this by shopping at the perimeter of the store

---

[11] "The NOVA Food Classification System" in *Food, Nutrition & Fitness I: The Digestion Journey Begins with Food Choices* by EduChange (with guidance from NUPENS), Sao Paulo: 2018. https://educhange.com/wp-content/uploads/2018/09/NOVA-Classification-Reference-Sheet.pdf.

where foods are, for the most part, found in their whole form. Avoiding packaged and convenience food in the aisles will help limit your intake of extra ingredients that add no purpose to your overall health and well-being. It will also help limit the intake of added fat and calories that so often come from convenience-type foods.

NON-STARCHY VEGETABLES

The trick to feeling satisfied is increasing your intake of ***free vegetables***! You can eat as many non-starchy vegetables as you want without having to worry about gaining weight. How often do you hear that you can eat as much of something as you want? As a dietitian, I can assure you it's not often! I encourage you to take advantage of this great opportunity to eat the colors of the rainbow. You have a wide variety of choices to make any meal interesting, and they come with some wonderful benefits. Non-starchy vegetables have been found to lower blood pressure, reduce the risk of cardiovascular disease and certain cancers, improve blood glucose control, and promote weight loss.[12] These vegetables are filled with fiber and disease-fighting compounds called antioxidants and phytochemicals, which all work together

---

[12] Joanne L. Slavin and Beate Lloyd, "Health Benefits of Fruits and Vegetables." *Advances in Nutrition* 3, no. 4 (July 2012): 506-516. doi: 10.3945/an.112.002154.

to keep the inside of the body in tip-top shape. They are also full of water, and when the fiber combines with the water in your stomach, it expands, and you feel full. Ultimately, that is how we want to feel when we are done with a meal.

The term "non-starchy" means these foods contain a relatively small amount of carbohydrates and have little to no caloric value. To be clear, little to no caloric value is not the same as little or no nutritional value. Examples of non-starchy vegetables can be found on page 207-208 of this book. Try and choose fresh vegetables whenever possible. If that cannot be done, then choose frozen vegetables that are not in a sauce and have no added salt. This will help control calories coming from the high-fat sauces. Many canned vegetables now have a no-salt-added option and often contain as little as ten mg of sodium. If you are using canned vegetables that contain sodium, rinse them under the faucet for a minute or two before preparing them. Just from rinsing, you can remove up to twenty-two percent of the salt from canned food.[13]

If you are not fond of many vegetables, take a moment to

---

[13] D.B. Haytowitz, "Effect of draining and rinsing on the sodium and water-soluble vitamin content of canned vegetables." Nutrient Data Laboratory, Beltsville Human Nutrition Research Center, Beltsville, MD. https://www.ars.usda.gov/ARSUserFiles/80400525/articles/eb11_drainedveg.pdf.

think about the last time you have eaten them. Our tastes change considerably over time, and what we do not like as a child may not be the same for us as adults. Challenge yourself to try one new non-starchy vegetable a week. You may find this opens your world to a lot more variety, which is one of the keys to optimal health. You owe it to yourself to give it a try. I think you will be pleasantly surprised!

WATER

Seventy percent of our body is comprised of water. The body requires water to function properly. I cannot stress enough the importance of consuming adequate amounts of water. Water helps to:

- regulate body temperature.
- transport nutrients and oxygen to the cells of the body.
- control blood pressure and heart rate.
- lubricate joints.
- promote optimal gastrointestinal function[14] .

While you want to ensure sufficient fluid intake for hydration, there is another important reason to focus on water as your main

---

[14] "Water and Healthier Drinks," Healthy Weight, Nutrition, and Physical Activity, Center for Disease Control and Prevention, last modified January 12, 2021, https://www.cdc.gov/healthywater/drinking/nutrition/index.html

beverage. The more you expose your palate to sweet foods and beverages, the more you will crave sweet foods and beverages. Part of this process of dietary change is to break the sometimes-constant desire for sweets. One way to accomplish this goal is to increase your intake of water and decrease your intake of sugary beverages, including diet drinks. While diet drinks will not cause weight gain, they do have the effect of keeping us wanting more sweet treats.

If you wish to have a diet beverage, limit it to mealtimes. This way, the other foods you consume at the meal will balance out the sweet taste of the diet drink. In between meals, keep your fluid intake to water and occasionally unsweetened iced tea. Aim for six to eight cups of water daily. Keep in mind that water can come in the form of other beverages as well as food. You can get twenty-five percent of your fluid needs met through the foods you eat. That is just another great reason to increase your intake of water-packed fruits and vegetables! Limiting caffeinated beverages to one eight-ounce glass a day is also beneficial[15].

MY FIRST VISIT WITH JANET

You remember our friend Janet from the last chapter, where she decided that today was the day that she was going to

---

[15] Isabelle Guelinckx et al., "Contribution of Water from Food and Fluids to Total Water Intake: Analysis of a French and UK Population Surveys." *Nutrients* 8, no. 10 (2016): 630. doi:10.3390/nu8100630.

change her life. She visited her GP, and the doctor put her in touch with me so that I could help her start her weight loss journey. As I told you before, I always start a meeting with a new patient with a question: What are you hoping to gain from this visit? Janet told me that she was hoping to regain her health and take control of her relationship with food. We talked about how that's a fantastic goal because the power is in her hands, and she can wield it. Now that we had some terrific intentions in mind, we could get down to work!

First, as I talked about in the last chapter, Janet would take a food log home with her--it would be her job over the next few days to measure everything she normally eats in a day. I told her, "It's important that you record everything you eat for a couple of days. Right now, it's not about trying to reduce intake; it's about figuring out your habits so that we can assess the best ways to help you take control."

She said, "I think I might be embarrassed to admit what I eat. I hate it when people watch how much I'm eating at a meal. I sometimes snack in the car when I'm doing my errands and then throw the wrappers away before my husband can see what I ate."

I reassured her, "This isn't for making judgments about you; it's for collecting data so that I can help you as much as possible. I am really happy that you've decided to take better care of yourself, and I want to help you succeed." She was reluctant but agreed to make an honest record of her food intake for the next three days.

"Next," I said, "we're going to calculate your body weight." She groaned audibly. "Again, it's just more information, Janet," I assured her. "We both know that you aren't the weight you want to be, so there won't be any shocks to know you're overweight now."

Janet took off her shoes (hey, she wasn't born in those shoes!) and stepped onto my scale. Her weight came up to 185 pounds. I measured her height next, and she came in at five feet five inches. These would be the numbers we would use to calculate her ideal body weight (IBW), adjusted body weight (ABW), and daily caloric needs (DCN) when she came back to see me after three days of food tracking.

Now you're going to put yourself into Janet's shoes (but you don't have to weigh them!). Weigh yourself, wearing an outfit that you can wear consistently for your weigh-ins (if you have the luxury of privacy, feel free to wear your birthday suit). Note this weight down because it's the starting point for your journey of transformation. Next to that, write your height in feet and inches. Finally, for the next three days, I'd like you to use the chart below to track your food intake. When you're all done with that, meet me at Chapter Three, and we will get started on your own calculations and the decisions you'll need to make to begin your empowered journey to weight loss and better health.

DATE	WEIGHT	HEIGHT
TIME	FOOD	AMOUNT CONSUMED

CHAPTER THREE: YOU'RE IN CONTROL

Sometimes, it feels like it's too much work to take control of your health and food choices. Like any new skill, it takes some time to get used to using the tools and establishing lasting habits. In this chapter, you will learn to make choices that empower you to prioritize your health and establish good patterns that lead to long-term success. In the last chapter, you delved into some of the facets of your relationship with food. To get ready for the work you'll do in this chapter, I'd like you to think about:

- What was it like to track your food intake? What sorts of feelings did it bring up? Did you enjoy being mindful of your food? Was it frustrating?
- What did you find surprising about your food intake log?
- What patterns did you notice about your daily consumption? Do you find that you are hungry at predictable times? Did you notice foods that triggered you to want more? Did eating certain foods make you want to eat other foods with them (For example: did eating chips after dinner make you want something sweet? Did having toast make you want to add butter and jam?)
- What are your go-to meals?
- What do you eat when you are busy, stressed, happy, tired?
- How did it feel to weigh yourself? Do you have lingering

feelings from past experiences of weighing in? Were you surprised by the number on the scale?

- Do you feel hopeful?

CALCULATING BODY WEIGHT

Stepping on the scale can be a tough thing to do. Sometimes, facing the number that looks back at us can be daunting or depressing. But like Janet, you already know that you aren't at your optimal weight today, and measuring the difference between where you are now and where you want to be is a big step toward achieving your goals. When I work with a client, it's my job to determine the body weight necessary to compute the appropriate number of calories to achieve that client's weight loss goal. There are different ways professionals do this. I use a formula for what is termed "adjusted body weight." Ideal body weight is sometimes used, but I prefer adjusted body weight because it generates a more realistic weight with which to calculate an individual's calorie needs.

Understand that the ideal or adjusted body weight you determine is not necessarily the weight you will achieve. It is the weight you will ultimately be aiming for. Many clients are sometimes concerned that the adjusted body weight is too low and they will never be able to attain that weight loss. The purpose behind the adjusted body weight is simply to gauge the number of calories needed to lose weight to move you in the right direction.

It does not mean that it is or should be a person's final weight goal.

There are many factors that affect weight loss and how many pounds an individual will lose. I suggest that my clients attempt a weight loss of ten percent of their present body weight as a practical place to start. For example, if the person weighs 180 pounds, they would be looking to lose approximately eighteen to twenty pounds in their initial weight loss effort. Research demonstrates that losing as little as seven to ten percent of your present body weight is the point where an individual starts to see significant health gains -- improvements in blood pressure, cholesterol, and/or blood glucose.[16] You are not limited to losing only ten percent of your initial weight, but setting and achieving small goals upfront will help provide the impetus to continue (we will learn more about how to set achievable goals in a later chapter). One of the dangers of setting our goals too high is the disappointment we might feel if we are unable to reach these higher goals. Disappointment can often be misinterpreted as failure if we are not mindful of our thoughts. This, in turn, can lead to giving up altogether.

The following formulas will help you to calculate your

---

[16] Donna H. Ryan and Sarah Ryan Yockey, "Weight Loss and Improvement in Comorbidity: Differences at 5%, 10%, 15%, and Over." *Current Obesity Reports* 6, no. 2 (2017): 187-194. doi:10.1007/s13679-017-0262-y.

adjusted body weight. The first step is to determine what the individual's **Ideal Body Weight (IBW)** should be. There are different formulas for men and women:[17]

> **IBW for men** is 106 pounds for the first five feet in height and 6 pounds for every inch over five feet.
>
> For example, if a man is five feet ten inches tall, his IBW would be calculated as follows:
>
> (One hundred and six pounds for the first five feet) + (ten inches x six pounds per inch over five feet) = **166 pounds**
>
> **IBW for women** is 100 pounds for the first five feet in height and 5 pounds for every inch over five feet.
>
> For example, if a woman is five feet four inches tall, her IBW would be calculated as follows:
>
> (100 pounds for the first five feet) + (four inches x five pounds per inch over five feet) = **120 pounds**

The next formula we need to use is the **Adjusted Body Weight (ABW)** formula to determine the weight we will use to calculate

---

[17] Courtney M. Peterson et al., "Universal equation for estimating ideal body weight and body weight at any BMI". *The American Journal of Clinical Nutrition* 103, no. 5. (2016): 1197-1203. doi:10.3945/ajcn.115.121178. Published correction appears in *The American Journal of Clinical Nutrition* 105, no. 3 (2017): 772.

calories. ABW formula is the same for both men and women:[18]

Present body weight – IBW = _____ x .25 (twenty five percent) = ____ + IBW

For example, if a woman weighs 180 pounds and is five feet four inches, we would do the following:

180 (present BW) – 120 (IBW) = 60 x .25 = 15 + 120 (IBW) = 135 pounds.

The ABW for this person is 135 pounds, and that is the number used to calculate calories needed to *promote* weight loss.

BODY MASS INDEX

I really had to consider whether or not to add information on BMI in this book as it has become a very controversial topic. There are two camps when it comes to BMI: those who feel it's useful and those who downright loathe it. I fall in the first camp. It is my professional opinion that BMI holds a useful place in the world of weight management. BMI is a simple tool to tell you if you are an appropriate weight for your height. That is it. It does not tell you if you are healthy. It is not a measure of one's blood glucose levels; it cannot tell you if your blood pressure is elevated,

---

[18] Gail Morrison and Lisa Hark, *Medical Nutrition and Disease: A Case-Based Approach.* (Cambridge, Massachusetts: Blackwell Science, 1996), 28.

and it can't diagnose you with cardiovascular disease. You need to have the appropriate blood work and other tests done to determine your overall health status. Somewhere along the line, a spin was put on it as if it was created as a measure of one's health, so let me repeat, **it is not.** While it is true that the proportion of lean muscle mass and fat, as well as bone density, differ from person to person, BMI *generally works well for the average individual.* BMI may not be accurate if you are a professional basketball player like Detroit Piston's Ben Wallace in his prime. It may not even be appropriate for a retired Ben Wallace since he still may have more lean muscle mass as an older individual than the average person. What we need to think about is that most of us, even with regular exercise, will never achieve the amount of lean muscle mass that a professional athlete does. If you have achieved that, then you would probably not be reading this book right now.

This is where I think BMI becomes an issue for people: we don't like what it is trying to convey. We don't like the words that are associated with it. It triggers a negative reaction inside of us based on the beliefs we have created around our weight. If something about BMI is triggering you, ask yourself why. BMI categorizes weight into normal, overweight, and obese. Does the name of the category you fall in feel offensive? Then, change the name. Categorize BMI as red, white, and blue. If you fall into the white or blue category, maybe you would benefit from weight loss.

I myself use BMI to keep myself in check. As the years have passed, I have found myself at the high end of normal. Then, my doctor's office measured my height, and I found myself one inch shorter than I had been a few years back. The loss of height didn't bother me as much as the fact that losing that one inch pushed my BMI over the normal threshold into overweight. To be honest, that didn't feel good to me. However, it made me want to get back into the normal range. Without it, I might keep telling myself, "Oh, it's only one pound, or it's only five pounds. I'm only slightly in the overweight category". BMI makes it clear to me when I need to make changes. That is how I would suggest that you use it. Remember earlier when I said that food can't speak to your morals or worth? Neither can BMI. But it can help keep you in check.

Here's a BMI chart so that you can check out where you fit in:

BMI	19	20	21	22	23	24	25	26	27	28	29	30	31	32	33	34	35
Height									Weight In Pounds								
4'10"	91	96	100	105	110	115	119	124	129	134	138	143	148	153	158	162	167
4'11"	94	99	104	109	114	119	124	128	133	138	143	148	153	158	163	168	173
5'	97	102	107	112	118	123	128	133	138	143	148	153	158	163	168	174	179
5'1"	100	106	111	116	122	127	132	137	143	148	153	158	164	169	174	180	185
5'2"	104	109	115	120	126	131	136	142	147	153	158	164	169	175	180	186	191
5'3"	107	113	118	124	130	135	141	146	152	158	163	169	175	180	186	191	197
5'4"	110	116	122	128	134	140	145	151	157	163	169	174	180	186	192	197	204
5'5"	114	120	126	132	138	144	150	156	162	168	174	180	186	192	198	204	210
5'6"	118	124	130	136	142	148	155	161	167	173	179	186	192	198	204	210	216
5'7"	121	127	134	140	146	153	159	166	172	178	185	191	198	204	211	217	223
5'8"	125	131	138	144	151	158	164	171	177	184	190	197	203	210	216	223	230
5'9"	128	135	142	149	155	162	169	176	182	189	196	203	209	216	223	230	236
5'10"	132	139	146	153	160	167	174	181	188	195	202	209	216	222	229	236	243
5'11"	136	143	150	157	165	172	179	186	193	200	208	215	222	229	236	243	250
6'	140	147	154	162	169	177	184	191	199	206	213	221	228	235	242	250	258
6'1"	144	151	159	166	174	182	189	197	204	212	219	227	235	242	250	257	265
6'2"	148	155	163	171	179	186	194	202	210	218	225	233	241	249	256	264	272
6'3"	152	160	168	176	184	192	200	208	216	224	232	240	248	256	264	272	279
	Healthy Weight						Overweight					Obese					

Source: US Department of Health and Human Services, National Institutes of Health, National Health, Lung, and Blood Institute. The Clinical Guidelines on the Identification, Evaluation and Treatment of Overweight and Obesity in Adults: Evidence Report. September 1998 [NIH pub. No. 98-4083].

CALCULATING CALORIE NEEDS

Calculating daily caloric needs can be done in various ways. I often use the short methods for calculating energy needs. The following table illustrates the multiplication factor to use based on gender, age, activity level, and weight category for adults:[19]

Men, active women	15 kcal/lb. body weight
Most women, sedentary men, and adults over 55 years	13 kcal/lb. body weight
Sedentary women, obese adults	10 kcal/lb. body weight

Simply multiply the weight by either ten, thirteen, or fifteen (based on your personal information) to determine caloric needs for weight loss. For instance, if a woman's body weight or ABW weight is 135 pounds and she is sedentary or obese, we multiply ten x 135 = 1350 calories needed a day to maintain or promote weight loss. If a man's body weight or ABW is 166 pounds and he is obese, we multiply ten x 166 = 1660 calories needed for weight loss. If you prefer to avoid doing the math, you can simply go to your Meal Wheel and pick the calorie level you would like

---

[19] Sylvia Escott-Stump, *Nutrition and Diagnosis-Related Care, Seventh Edition.* (Baltimore, Maryland: Lippincott Williams & Wilkins, 2012), 608.

to try. Most women can lose weight following a 1200 - 1500 calorie meal plan, and men can usually lose weight safely following a 1500 - 1800 calorie plan.

I err on the lower side when I calculate daily calorie needs for my patients, as I find most people tend to underestimate their intake. This gives the individual some cushion; should they overconsume their calories a little bit, they will still be close to the recommended level. Also, keep in mind that some days, you may consume fewer calories and other days more. That is okay. The goal is to keep your chosen calorie level consistent from week to week.

CHECKING IN WITH JANET

Janet came back to my office with her food intake log. Before she handed it to me, she said, "I'm nervous about sharing this with you." I asked her what she was worried would happen when I went over the log with her, and she said, "I'm afraid you will judge me. I noticed when I started writing things down that I eat a lot of snacks after dinner, and I never realized what a half-cup portion of ice cream looks like. I always thought I was having a serving, but once I measured what I normally put into a bowl, I saw that I was really eating **three** servings at a time."

I assured Janet that the things she observed are things that everyone notices when they start to log what they actually eat. She wasn't weird or having an unusual experience. We usually underestimate our portion sizes for a lot of different reasons. We aren't really aware of how much a teaspoon, tablespoon, or cup really is, and we are constantly surrounded by restaurant portions that have crept up in size every year until they are enormous; some restaurant meals are five or six servings of food, presented to you on a single plate (and maybe even triggering your desire to be "good" and "clean your plate" --leftover feelings from childhood).

When I looked at Janet's log, it confirmed my suspicions. Her problems were the same as those of many of my clients: skipping meals (she wasn't a fan of breakfast and often just had a cup of coffee with half and half instead), outsized portions, and evening snacking. "Janet, this is fantastic. These are all problems that you can address with mindfulness. There's nothing here that you can't take control of."

I handed Janet a whiteboard marker. "Now, let's calculate your **ideal body weight (IBW), adjusted body weight (ABW), and daily caloric needs (DCN)**. These are the numbers that will give us all the information we need to get your journey to better health off to a great start."

Using the formula I described above, Janet started out by calculating her IBW. "It's been a while since I've done any math on the board," she joked, "or since I was my ideal weight. I'm five feet five inches, so," she wrote down 100 (the base weight for women's first five feet of height) and then took the remaining 5 inches over five feet and multiplied that by 5. 5x5=25, plus 100=

125. "Wow. My ideal weight is 125 pounds. That means I'm 60 pounds over my ideal."

I reminded her that the next step would be to *adjust* her body weight. We would multiply the 60 pounds by .25, giving us a total of 15 pounds of adjustment. Janet's adjusted body weight (ABW) would be 140 pounds.

"What do I do with that number? Is that what I'm trying to set as my final goal?"

I explained that we would set some goals and intentions soon. Right now, that number 140 would give us what we needed to figure out how many calories a day Janet should be consuming in order to support healthy and sustainable weight loss. Since Janet's BMI of 30.8 put her in the "obese" category, we chose the bottom box, giving us a 10kcal/lb of bodyweight number to add to our equation.

"Oh wow. I hate the word 'obese!' It makes me feel awful and judged. I knew I was overweight, but I guess I didn't realize how far it had gone." I saw tears shining in her eyes. "Janet, I'm sorry that the word upsets you, but it can only make you feel as bad as you let it. Knowing where you stand is very important to improving your health and supporting you in accomplishing your goals. Let's call it "Blue Zone" instead. You don't have to let words with negative associations keep you from what you want. We will work together to get you out of the Blue Zone and into the White. That will be our first goal."

Janet nodded her head. "Okay. You're right. If one of my kids let one word prevent them from achieving their goals, I'd tell them not to be silly. I can do this." She wrote: 140x10=1400 on the whiteboard. "So, if I'm eating 1,400 calories a day, I will be able to see progress toward weight loss? When you first explained the equations to me, I thought they sounded really intimidating, but it was pretty easy to do."

I explained that since she had mastered the formula, she'd be able to maintain a slow and steady pace toward her goals.

CHAPTER FOUR: USING THE MEAL WHEEL TO MAKE GREAT FOOD CHOICES

Maybe you've been wondering why this book is called *The Meal Wheel Method for Weight Management* since, so far, there haven't been any wheels in sight. The Meal Wheel is a tool I developed to help my clients make the best choices they can to support their path to health, to give their bodies what's needed to function and thrive, and to be happy and not feel deprived while doing it. Before you start out with this useful tool, I'd like you to consider how you feel about making this new commitment to yourself:

- What are the most successful commitments you've made in your life? (Think about family, education, career, romantic partnerships, mortgages, etc.). What keeps you on track to meet these commitments?
- What tradeoffs do you have to make to make these successful commitments work?
- What tradeoffs are you willing to make to improve your health? Will you limit the things you like? Are you willing to try new foods or kinds of exercise? What else?
- How do you imagine it will feel to be successful at losing weight and improving your health?
- What are the pros and cons of making this commitment to

yourself?

- How will you be accountable? Who do you think you should be accountable to? What would it feel like to be accountable to yourself?

FROM MEAL WHEEL TO MEAL PLAN

In the last chapter, you (and Janet) used the formulas to calculate your target number of calories to consume to support healthy weight loss. But where should those calories come from? While **mathematically,** it doesn't matter if you consume 1,400 calories of lean protein, complex carbohydrates, and fresh fruits and vegetables **or** 12 ½ servings of chocolate ice cream, **it matters a lot to your body.** Making smart choices in how you plan your meals to support your weight loss goals **and** give your body the fuel it needs to do its best work may seem daunting, but it is not very difficult once you get the hang of it. It can be challenging at the start, but you will get better with practice.

I start my patients with very basic meal plans. Then, we work our way up over time to more creative menus. In my opinion, meal planning is more about *how much* you eat rather than *what* you eat. The key is to properly portion out the foods you choose to eat and the beverages you drink. I will go through each calorie level and show you how to do meal planning in its most basic form. What may seem fundamental at first will provide you with a solid foundation on which to begin experimenting to develop more complicated meal plans on your own once you are comfortable with the general formula.

Try to follow my lead and attempt to create some simple meals of your own. I have included templates for each of the calorie levels to help you with your meal planning. They are located in Appendix C at the back of the book. Be sure to balance your meals by including carbohydrates, protein, and fat per your Meal Wheel options. Balancing your plate will help you feel full between meals and ensure you are meeting your basic nutrient requirements. If you are feeling hungry or want more food at a meal, use the foods on the Freebie pages 207-208—you may consume as much of those foods as you like without having to count them. The idea here is to decrease the intake of calorically dense foods and increase the intake of foods that are low in calories and packed with fiber and other valuable nutrients. You never have to feel hungry if you select the right foods!

Let's look at the Meal Wheel to understand how to use it. Side A of the Meal Wheel lists how much of each food group you can consume over the course of the day. For those of you who want to be more in control, Side A will permit you to make more choices on your own. This option provides the greatest amount of flexibility and will allow you to develop your meals any way you want. For instance, if you like more protein or carbohydrate at a certain meal, you can use it there. Side B does a lot of the work for you by separating the food into meals and directing you on how much food from each major food group to consume at each meal. I propose starting with Side B first since it is preset to ensure that your meals are balanced, and it will help you get used to the correct serving sizes. Meals should be consumed every four to five hours with an evening snack. Skipping meals is always discouraged. Include non-starchy vegetables all day!

Use your portion guide on pages 201-212 to understand how to measure each serving. All amounts in the portion guide are based on ***one serving***. In the next couple of sections, I will explain how to use both the portion guide and food label to determine a single portion.

Side A

1200 Calories
Non-starchy Vegetables
8 Carbohydrate Choices
5 oz Protein
3 Fat Choices
1300 Calories
Non-starchy Vegetables
9 Carbohydrate Choices
5 oz Protein
3 Fat Choices
1400 Calories
Non-starchy Vegetables
9 Carbohydrate Choices
6 oz Protein
4 Fat Choices
1500 Calories
Non-starchy Vegetables
10 Carbohydrate Choices
6 oz Protein
4 Fat Choices
1600 Calories
Non-starchy Vegetables
11 Carbohydrate Choices
6 oz Protein
5 Fat Choices
1700 Calories
Non-starchy Vegetables
11 Carbohydrate Choices
8 oz Protein
5 Fat Choices
1800 Calories
Non-starchy Vegetables
12 Carbohydrate Choices
8 oz Protein
5 Fat Choices

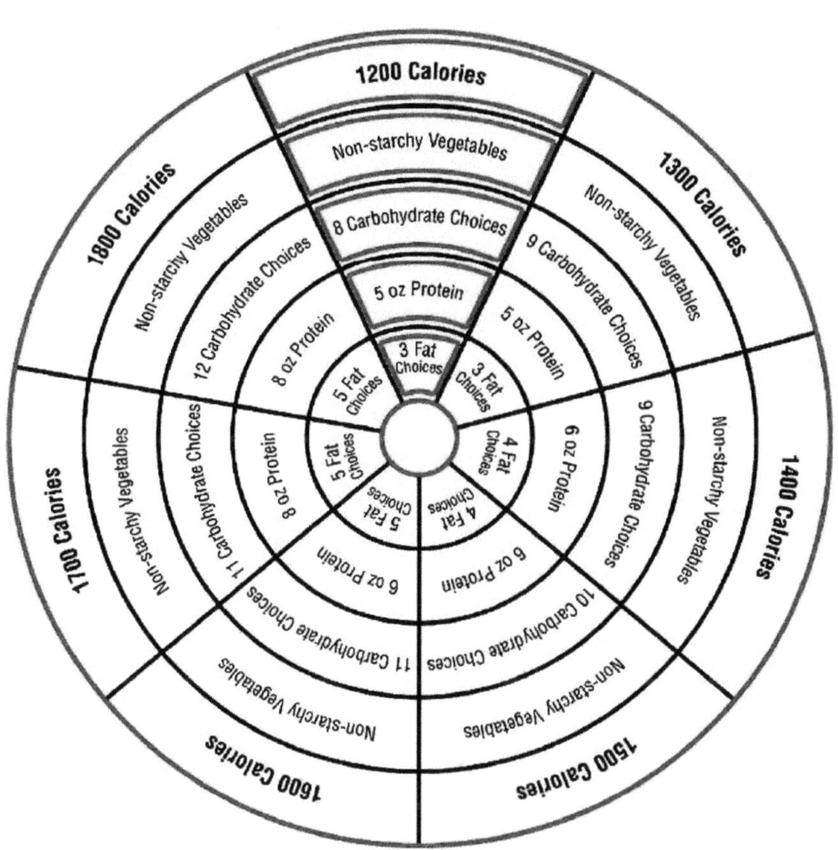

Side B

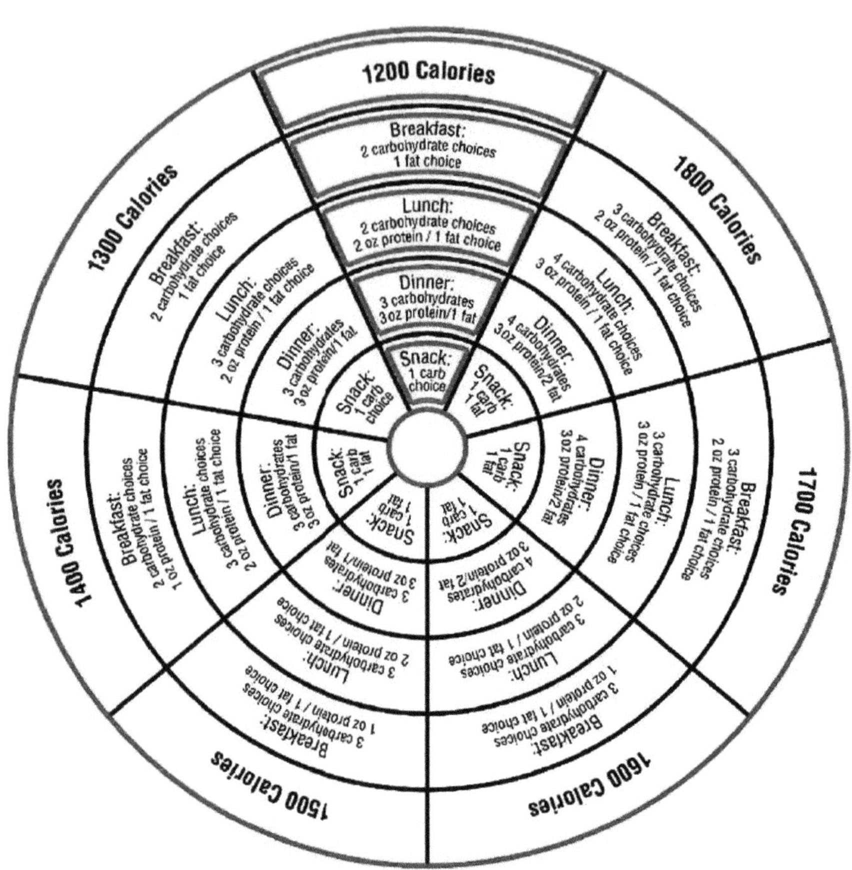

SERVING SIZES & GUIDELINES

While there are a lot of factors to managing your weight, portion control is, in my opinion, one of the most important. If you want to eat high-calorie food, you could offset the impact of the food on your diet by monitoring portion sizes. This is great news! Portion control allows you to consume foods that you enjoy in smaller quantities without "blowing" your entire diet. It is also a more realistic way to live and will help you create a healthier relationship with food.

I recall that many years ago, a friend of mine had lost some weight. We had both graduated from college and were trying to shed some of the freshman fifteen we'd gained. My first college degree was in business. I was not a dietitian at the time. I asked her how she did it, and she told me that she allowed herself to have small amounts of the foods she desired without feeling guilty. I decided to give it a try. What I found, over time, as I applied this way of thinking, was that I was naturally creating a sounder relationship with food. What happens when you are told you cannot have something? You probably want it more. By allowing myself to have some of the things I liked some of the time, I took away that feeling of lacking that people experience when they cut themselves off from food they enjoy. If I decide to consume fun food, I tend to be quite satisfied with a relatively small amount. I have gained an incredible sense of control over my eating habits just by changing my perception and surrendering to smaller portions. You will, too.

There are many factors that affect how much we eat. Consuming large portions of food may have come from the environment we grew up in ("clean your plate! There are folks starving in the world!"), or we may eat emotionally ("I had a lousy day, I deserve ice cream") or we may eat frequently in restaurants that serve 2, 3, or 4 servings on a single plate (it feels like getting your money's worth).

Learning how to use the portion section of the book, as well as how to read a food label, is an integral part of success with the Meal Wheel. Portion control is the foundation of this method of weight loss. The food label is the gold standard, and you should use it if one is available, as it will provide the most accurate information. The portion guidelines in the book will also be helpful, but they are more of an average of similar foods rather than an exact amount of a specific food. I will show you how to determine portions for all the macronutrients so that you'll be able to calculate serving sizes on your own. Please do not be discouraged by the single-serving amounts that you see. You may feel disappointed or even scared to decrease your food intake. Smaller portions of food will not harm you if you decrease the portions correctly. The upside to portion control is that you are not limited to one serving per meal. Once you get into the rhythm of more appropriate portions, you won't even miss the larger ones!

CARBOHYDRATE: BEYOND THE BASICS

One serving of carbohydrates is defined as fifteen grams of carbohydrates. All the carbohydrate foods listed in the portion guide are given in their ***single serving*** measurement and, when measured out, are equivalent to ***fifteen grams***. This number is important to know to help you keep within your carbohydrate recommendations at mealtimes. Let's look at some examples to see what fifteen grams of carbohydrates mean as part of a meal plan.[20]

If you choose a meal plan that allows for three carbohydrate choices per meal, then you get a total of forty-five grams of carbohydrate per meal because each carbohydrate choice equals fifteen grams of carbohydrate. Three servings and forty-five grams are just two different ways of saying the same thing. As shown in the Meal Wheel, three carbohydrate choices or forty-five grams look like this:

1 choice **or** 15 grams + 1 choice **or** 15 grams + 1 choice **or** 15 grams = 3 choices or 45 grams.

Using the portion guide in the book, you will find that each fifteen-

---

[20] "Carb Counting and Diabetes." American Diabetes Association. Accessed Jan. 15, 2015, https://www.diabetes.org/healthy-living/recipes-nutrition/understanding-carbs/carb-counting-and-diabetes.

gram choice can come from the same food: one-third cup brown rice (fifteen grams) + one-third cup brown rice (fifteen grams) + one-third cup brown rice (fifteen grams) = forty-five grams for a total of one cup of brown rice. Or, they can come from two different foods: one-third cup brown rice (fifteen grams) + one-third cup brown rice (fifteen grams) + one-half cup green peas (fifteen grams) = forty-five grams, for a meal that contains two-thirds cup of brown rice and one-half cup of green peas. Or, they can come from three different food choices: one-third cup brown rice (fifteen grams) + one-half cup black beans (fifteen grams) + one-half cup corn (fifteen grams) = forty-five grams.

The beautiful part of this is that you can mix and match your foods any way you like to get what you desire. It might take some time to get used to this system and to measure out your portions. You may not be eating the same amount as previously, but these are the changes that will help you lose weight. As a dietitian, it still shocks me how little food we actually need to be healthy. We think we need more because that is what we are used to eating. Once you compare what you are presently eating to what I am asking you to do, it will become evident why you will lose weight.

If you choose foods that contain a lot of added sugar, your portions of food become even smaller. This is never a good thing if you like feeling full! People feel good when they consume a certain volume of food. It keeps us from feeling deprived. Keep this in mind as you make your daily choices. For example, if you decide to have a twelve-ounce regular soda with your lunch, that equals roughly thirty-nine to forty-two grams of carbohydrate alone from the soda! You would be consuming between two and a half and three servings. Recall that each serving is fifteen grams, so you would divide the total forty-two by fifteen to get about three servings just from your beverage. Depending on which calorie level you choose to follow, there may not be enough carbohydrates left for the bread to make a sandwich and a snack bag of baked potato chips. Sugary beverages are never a good choice because they "use up" all of your carbohydrate servings for a meal. If you were to drink water instead, you would still have forty-five grams of carbohydrates for food. That could translate into two slices of whole grain bread for thirty grams of carbohydrates and either a small piece of fruit or a four-ounce yogurt for fifteen grams, to bring your total to forty-five grams of carbohydrates. You could even consume a small side salad. Experience has taught me you are much more likely to feel full if your calories come from food rather than from beverages. Don't forget whole foods such as whole grains and fruit contain a lot of fiber and water, which makes us feel satiated and less likely to snack on empty calories between meals. Supplement meals with freebie non-starchy vegetables, and the amount of food you will be able to consume while keeping your calorie intake down will astound you!

A balanced diet will always require some form of carbohydrate at all meals. It would be a good idea to make a list of the carbohydrate foods you regularly consume and identify the carbohydrates that are coming from empty calories (processed snack foods and refined carbohydrates). From there, make another list of healthy carbohydrate substitutes. Use that list when you create your menus to help keep the nutrient-poor carbohydrate intake to a minimum. If you (or Janet or any of my patients) think that they do not like nutrient-rich food, it may be that they are not in the habit of making the conscious choice to eat these types of food. Once making a healthy choice becomes your habit, you will be on your way to losing weight.

PROTEIN: BEYOND THE BASICS

One serving or one ounce of protein is equivalent to seven grams of protein. You will need between six and eight ounces of protein daily. This equates to about fifty grams of protein a day for women and sixty grams a day for men to meet their basic protein requirements. Since we obtain protein from a variety of foods, there should be little concern with inadequate intake.

The distribution of protein throughout the day could look like this:

Women–six ounces of protein:

- Breakfast: one-quarter cup cottage cheese (one-ounce equivalent)
- Lunch: one and a half ounces of turkey breast and one-half

ounce of cheese (two ounces)

- Dinner: three ounces of chicken breast

Men–eight ounces of protein:

- Breakfast: two eggs (two-ounce equivalents)
- Lunch: one and a half ounces of chicken breast and one-half ounce of cheese (two ounces)
- Dinner: four ounces of pork tenderloin

The ounces can be split up any way you like over the course of the day. The important point is to not exceed the number of ounces suggested by the Meal Wheel per day. Every ounce you exceed is extra calories you don't need! The more calories you consume above what you require to lose weight, the slower the weight loss or the less weight you will lose.

People consume a great deal of calories from the protein they eat because most protein sources contain naturally occurring fat. That means that if you were to eat two extra ounces of protein a day from a high-fat source like cheese, that would equal an additional two hundred calories for that day (one hundred calories per ounce of high-fat protein)! Choose lean meats and cheeses in addition to staying within the recommended parameters. Always remember, the higher the fat content of the protein, the higher the calories per ounce.

FAT: BEYOND THE BASICS

Fat contains five grams and about forty-five calories per serving. Your intake of fat *must* be limited to control calories. This is probably the easiest area for people to overeat without realizing it. This happens because we don't understand what a serving is—most fat servings are relatively small.

Some examples of servings of fat are:

- Butter—one teaspoon (45 calories)
- Olive oil—one teaspoon (40 calories)
- Peanut butter—one teaspoon (31 calories)
- Almonds—9 almonds (63 calories) *

*You might remember that when he was in office, President Obama was reported as eating a nightly snack of seven almonds.[21] This idea shows up in the film *The Devil Wears Prada*, too, where, if we pay close attention, we notice a woman preparing her breakfast and carefully measuring out her almonds. Both of these examples were about poking fun, but actually, they are both spot-on for mindful consumption of fat. A portion of romaine lettuce that matches the 40 calories in that teaspoon of olive oil, for example, is **5 CUPS!** It's not that fats are "bad" and lettuce is

---

[21] "Obama After Dark: The Precious Hours Alone," *The New York Times*, July 2, 2016, https://www.nytimes.com/2016/07/03/us/politics/obama-after-dark-the-precious-hours-alone.html.

“good”—rather, it’s about knowing what you’re consuming and how it will impact your weight loss goals.

According to the Meal Wheel, most women should keep their fat intake to no more than three or four servings, and most men only need four or five servings per day! Butter, margarine, and mayonnaise are each one teaspoon per serving. Almonds, cashews, and peanuts fall between six to ten nuts per serving. When you consider the Meal Wheel recommendations for added fat a day, it doesn’t leave much wiggle room! Where is the fat in your diet coming from?

If you are using the Meal Wheel to follow a 1,200-calorie diet, fat servings per meal would look like this based on three servings of fat a day:

- Breakfast: one teaspoon of butter
- Lunch: one tablespoon of salad dressing
- Dinner: one teaspoon of olive oil for cooking

The problem with the plan above is not only that we usually use more than one teaspoon of butter on our toast, but we also may be eating two slices of toast, using cream in our coffee, and possibly having two or three slices of bacon while consuming an egg breakfast. That breakfast is equivalent to six or seven servings of added fat—double what is recommended for the entire day! Obviously, it continues as the day progresses because we may use one tablespoon or more of salad dressing on our salad and mayonnaise on our sandwich at lunch. We haven't even included dinner yet! You don't get much value when it comes to added fat. Try to choose lower-fat options whenever possible. Use low-fat mayonnaise on your sandwich or balsamic vinegar on your salad so you can use your other added fats where they make you happiest. Always use measuring spoons, leveled off, for accuracy.

You must consider, as well, the types of foods you are choosing to consume. If you are keeping within your carbohydrate recommendations but are choosing foods that are produced with added fat, such as baked goods, you will overconsume calories for which the Meal Wheel does not account. Added fat can be sneaky. It often shows up where we don't expect it, or we don't always look for it. Keep an eye on this crafty nutrient to ensure weight loss.

THE NUTRITION FACTS LABEL

The Food and Drug Administration (FDA) requires most packaged and processed foods to have a nutrition facts label.[22] This ensures that the food industry complies with specific requirements pertaining to nutrient content claims and health messages. This label is a wonderful tool that can assist in making

---

[22] "Label 1." U.S. Food and Drug Administration. https://www.fda.gov/food/food-labeling-nutrition/nutrition-facts-label-images-download.

informed choices as well as aid in meal planning. Becoming familiar with how to use it properly is essential to follow a healthy diet. Reading and understanding the nutrition facts label is much the same as reading and understanding a recipe. You can't just go to the top of a recipe and start cooking. Seasoned experienced chefs recommend that you read the entire recipe first, then gather your ingredients, and then prepare everything before you even start to cook. This is similar to reading the nutrition facts label in that you need to take your time, look at the whole label, and then focus on the key bits of information that you need to prepare your plate. If a recipe calls for one cup of flour, then that is what you would measure out. If your Meal Wheel calls for one serving of carbohydrate then that is what you will measure out.

Although it's important for you to understand how to use the information on the nutrition facts label to make healthy food choices and to portion foods out to fit into your meal plan, I also encourage you to choose whole foods that don't come in a box with a label. The foods I am referring to are fresh, minimally processed, or unprocessed and can typically be found along the perimeter of the store. Your focus should be on fresh vegetables, fruit, whole grains, lean protein, and low-fat dairy. In most food stores, it is in the aisles of the store where you find the foods that are processed and contain many extra ingredients that are not very good for our bodies. They often contain salt, fat, sugar, stabilizers, and preservatives. With processed food, you will need to pay close attention to the nutrition facts label.

Earlier, I introduced you to the portion section of the book as a means of determining single-serving amounts. Using the nutrition facts label is another way to do that. The food label is the gold standard and, if available, should be used. It contains the most accurate information and will help you determine the appropriate amount. Learn to use the nutrition facts label to your benefit. It's a treasure trove for folks who want to take control of their relationship with food. Let's take a look!

Nutrition Facts

8 servings per container
Serving size **2/3 cup (55g)**

Amount per serving
Calories **230**

	% Daily Value*
Total Fat 8g	**10%**
Saturated Fat 1g	**5%**
Trans Fat 0g	
Cholesterol 0mg	**0%**
Sodium 160mg	**7%**
Total Carbohydrate 37g	**13%**
Dietary Fiber 4g	**14%**
Total Sugars 12g	
Includes 10g Added Sugars	**20%**
Protein 3g	
Vitamin D 2mcg	10%
Calcium 260mg	20%
Iron 8mg	45%
Potassium 235mg	6%

* The % Daily Value (DV) tells you how much a nutrient in a serving of food contributes to a daily diet. 2,000 calories a day is used for general nutrition advice.

The label lists nutrients found in one serving of the food. The serving size on the label is not a suggested amount to consume. It is the amount of food that people are likely to eat. You must keep in mind that if you have more than one serving of the food, all of the numbers on the label will increase, including the calories. Always start at the top of the label with servings per container and serving size. It can be very enlightening to find that the food item you purchased contains multiple servings—especially if the package is small. Label facts are always based on a two-thousand-calorie diet. However, the information on the label can be used by everyone, even if your calorie needs are less than two thousand. Recognize that energy needs vary from person to person because they are based on an individual's gender, height, weight, and level of physical activity. The Meal Wheel uses general calorie levels that promote weight loss in both women and men.

In the FDA [23] example food label above, we find that there are eight servings per container. Each serving is a two-thirds-cup portion that contains 230 calories. If you choose to have two servings, the equivalent of one and one-third cups, your caloric intake increases to 460 calories from just one food. Calories continue to increase if you consume other foods along with this one. That seems pretty straightforward. When we take a closer look at this label, we will also find some interesting yet little-

[23] Ibid.

known tidbits.

The label includes information on all of the macronutrients, but for the purpose of getting started, we are going to center our attention on total carbohydrates from which the majority of our calories are derived. Again, you will first look at the serving size and decide how much of the food you plan on eating. If you decide to have one serving, you would measure out two-thirds of a cup. Next, go to ***total carbohydrates*** and determine how many grams are in the two-thirds cup portion. The label states thirty-seven grams in this example. So, how many servings of carbohydrates are you actually consuming if you eat a two-thirds-cup portion? According to the definition, one serving of carbohydrates equals fifteen grams. You must divide thirty-seven by fifteen to identify how many servings you are actually receiving. In this case, you would be consuming two and a half servings. If your total carbohydrates, according to your Meal Wheel, allow for three servings (or forty-five grams) you are good to go. If the Meal Wheel proposes thirty grams of carbohydrates per meal, then this portion, even though it is only one serving of this particular food according to the label, will cause you to over consume carbohydrates at the meal. Likewise, if you consume two servings of this food, your total carbohydrate coming from this particular food will be seventy-four grams or five servings. Of course, this assumes that this food is the only source of carbohydrates at the meal. That's why, if you can learn to stay within the carbohydrate servings suggested by the Meal Wheel and stay within the guidelines suggested for protein and fat, you will be on your way to losing weight.

It's quite easy to overeat if you only follow the servings on the label. Labels provide correct information, but they do not explain how to interpret and use that information. It is easy to consume more than you need. Let's break down a normal breakfast meal to show you a real-life example of how we overeat on a regular basis and don't realize it because it doesn't look like that much food.

- 1 ½ cups of a frosted wheat cereal = ~66 grams of carbohydrate or ~4 ½ servings
- 1 cup of 2% milk = approximately 15 grams of carbohydrate or 1 serving
- 4 ounces of orange juice = 15 grams of carbohydrate or 1 serving
- Total carbohydrates at this meal = 96 gram or about 6 ½ servings

Cold cereal with milk and orange juice does not appear to be a lot of food. In terms of volume, it's not. The dilemma here is that if you are trying to keep your carbohydrates to forty-five grams per meal, you would need to cut the volume of this meal in half. So, what are your options? You could choose a cereal that contains no added sugar and get a larger quantity of food with fewer carbohydrates and fewer calories. Or, you could consume a completely different breakfast. Choosing foods that are naturally lower in carbohydrates per serving, such as two slices of peanut butter toast with a small banana, provides more volume.

The big question I am usually asked is "*What* can I eat?" To me, the more important question is *how much* can I eat of the foods I choose? If you are going over your budget for carbohydrates at a meal, try keeping the same foods you are used to eating and measuring them using the Meal Wheel portions. Ask yourself if you can be happy with this amount. Will you make it to the next meal without being hungry? If the answer to these questions is "no," then you need an alternate plan. Try a different food. See what would happen if you added a piece of fruit. You could have one and a half cups of a plain unsweetened cereal with a half cup of low-fat milk and half of a small banana for your forty-five grams of carbohydrates with a lot fewer calories. Could you be happy with that amount of food? Play around with different meal ideas to learn about what food combinations will be most fulfilling for you. Only you can decide what works for you.

It's critical to point out that there really is no place for sugar-sweetened anything if you are trying to lose weight. The empty calories that come from refined sugar are not worth it. This includes juice. Juice is disguised as being healthy because it comes from fruit. While it is true that juice contains some nutrients, from a carbohydrate standpoint it is still like drinking soda. Eating a piece of fruit is just as tasty and full of fiber to help fill your belly.

The breakfast example I presented did not contain fat. Be reminded that dietary fat is usually a significant source of calories. If you decided to have an egg breakfast, as an alternative, that might include buttered toast, sausage or bacon, and coffee with creamer. It may be easier to control the carbohydrate intake for an egg breakfast, but then the fat intake becomes the complicating factor. Consider the advice given by the Meal Wheel in regard to fat and protein recommendations. As you can see, we need to approach weight loss in a well-rounded manner because all foods increase calories. All foods count.

To recap, there are two ways to determine servings: the portion guide and the FDA nutrition facts food label. If a label isn't available, you can use the portion section of this book to help you. The portion section simply lists all foods in their single serving amount. You just need to select your foods and measure them based on the information provided in the portion guide. The more educated you are about the food you put into your body, and the more engaged you are with your food habits, the better off you will be.

MENU PLANNING: PULLING IT TOGETHER

The next few sections are dedicated to menu planning. In the first section, you will master how to analyze your initial food record and compare it to the Meal Wheel calorie level of your choice. This activity will provide insight into your present dietary habits and will direct your focus on where to make relevant intake adjustments. You will gain knowledge and knowledge is power.

In the second section, you will begin to create your own menus. I assembled some basic menus as a reference and included the food portions to support you in this process. There are blank templates located in Appendix C on pages 213-224. The templates should be chosen based on an appropriate calorie level. Using these convenient forms will take most of the guesswork out of meal planning and organize the material obtained from your Meal Wheel. Begin by selecting the foods you wish to consume, looking them up in the portion guide (or using a food label if one is available), measure them out, and plug them in. It's as easy as that!

When constructing your menus, don't leave anything out. If the Meal Wheel calls for three servings of carbohydrates, then include food for all three servings. Ensuring adequate food intake will boost metabolism and maximize satiety. Once the initial leg work is done and the menus are created, I suggest keeping them in a binder. This will provide you with access to a variety of different meals at any time.

FOOD RECALL ANALYSIS

Remember the food recall you did at the beginning of our adventure? Now is when you pull that out to compare your current eating habits to the recommended servings of carbohydrates, fat, and protein suggested by your Meal Wheel plan. Let's look together at our previous example:

TIME	FOOD	AMOUNT	EQUIVALENTS
9:30 a.m.	Eggs, scrambled in butter	2 2 tsp	2 oz. of medium-fat protein 2 fat servings
	Scrapple	3 oz.	3 oz. of high-fat protein
	Home fries	1 cup	2 carbohydrate servings 1 fat serving
	Rye bread toasted	2 slices	2 carbohydrate servings
	Butter	1 Tbsp.	3 fat servings
	Tomato juice	8 oz.	Freebie (but high in sodium!)
	Coffee	12 oz.	Freebie
	Creamer	2 Tbsp.	1 fat serving
	Artificial sweetener	1 packet	Freebie
	MEAL TOTALS		**5 oz. protein** **4 carbohydrate servings** **7 fat servings**
12:30	Mixed greens	2 cups	Freebie

p.m.			
	Grilled chicken breast	4 oz.	4 oz. of very lean protein
	Caesar salad dressing	¼ cup	4 fat servings
	Diet soda	12 oz.	Freebie
	MEAL TOTALS		**0 carbohydrate servings** **4 oz. of protein** **4 fat servings**
7:30 p.m.	Wheat pasta, cooked	2 cups	6 carbohydrate servings
	Marinara sauce	¾ cup	Freebie (depends on the sauce)
	Meatballs, brand x	4 oz.	4 oz. medium-high-fat protein
	Salad	1 cup	Freebie
	Ranch dressing	¼ cup	4 fat servings
	Diet soda	12 oz.	Freebie
	MEAL TOTALS		**6 carbohydrate servings** **4 oz. protein** **4+ fat servings**
8:30 p.m.	Ice cream	1 cup	2 carbohydrate servings

			2 fat servings
	SNACK TOTALS		**2 carbohydrate servings** **2 fat servings**

Now let's take the total carbohydrate, protein, and fat from the initial food record and compare it to the 1,400-calorie Meal Wheel suggestion. Your comparison will be based on the calorie level that you choose.

MY USUAL DAILY INTAKE	**1,400 CALORIES PER MEAL WHEEL**
12 carbohydrate choices (4-0-6-2)	9 carbohydrate choices (2-3-3-1)
13 oz. of protein (varying fat content)	6 oz. of lean protein
17 fat choices	4 fat choices

What I have done here (I suggest you do as well now that you know how to calculate serving sizes) is go back and put the foods from my initial food recall into their single-serving amounts. I then totaled up all of the single servings so that I could compare the totals to my Meal Wheel calorie choice breakdown. The "usual intake" totals are not so unusual. In fact, this is typical of what I see. No one sets out to intentionally overeat. However, if you do not understand what the appropriate portions are for you to lose weight, you will continuously overeat.

The takeaway here is that this person's usual intake far exceeds 2000 calories a day with too many calories coming from each main food group. The calories coming from carbohydrates are actually the most reasonable and the closest to the Meal Wheel suggestion. The number of calories coming from fat and protein is the real dilemma. We could decrease the caloric intake by 500 calories a day (the equivalent of 3500 calories, or one pound a week) if we just get the fat intake down to the suggested four servings a day. This is why I consistently caution you to monitor the fat intake, as a little adds up to be a lot!

Remember to be mindful of your protein intake as well. Lots of folks think of protein as "free" so they can eat a lot of it. They believe that because it is not carbohydrate, then it is fine to eat--regardless of the amount. The trouble with this way of rationalizing is how easy it is to consume too many calories. You will certainly do better if you make low-fat protein choices because the fat content of the meat products we ingest adds a significant number of calories to the diet. Be reminded that the purpose of the food recall is to note poor habits with an eye toward changing them. Now that you have the knowledge and training about portions and serving sizes, you can identify where you have been out of balance in the past and are now ready to implement these changes.

CHECKING IN WITH JANET

Janet started her journey with a 1,400-calorie-a-day target. She kept up with her meal logging, and began measuring all of her portions (she said, "I just keep the measuring spoons out on the counter. No reason to put them back because I use them all the time and seeing them reminds me to use them!"), and made an effort to shift some of the calories she usually ate in the evening for snacks to give her body some fuel to start with in the morning in the form of breakfast. When she came back to see me after two weeks, we had a lot to talk about.

"It's been taking up a lot of my attention to measure and track all of my food. Robin, does it get any easier?"

I promised her that like any skill, the more she practiced, the less difficult she would find it. "That doesn't mean it will be easy. You are developing habits you'll want to keep for a lifetime. That means you will practice them every day. Some days it will be easy and some days it will be hard. But if you keep your goals in mind, you'll be able to remember that attaining your goals is worth the tradeoffs."

"At our last visit, you gave me some specific instructions, and I made those my goals for these last two weeks: less snacking, more tracking, and starting the day with breakfast. I think I did a really good job of accomplishing those goals. How do I set a long-term weight loss goal? In other words, how will I know when I've accomplished what I've set out to do?"

"Ah, Janet! I love this part," I said, "this is where you get to decide your own terms for how you will succeed. You choose the goal, and you are empowered to accomplish it. Let's get started."

CHAPTER FIVE: GOALS (FOOD, EXERCISE, STRESS, LIFE)

Now that you have all the information you need to make informed choices about how to give your body the fuel it needs to survive and thrive while you are losing excess weight, it's time to set some goals. I believe in setting a combination of goals--measurable, attainable goals that you can set for both *short-term* and *long-term* success. Deciding how much you will exercise, what foods you will eat, and how you will support your mental health while you are losing and maintaining weight are all important goals to set, so that you are constantly moving forward, and so that you can measure and celebrate your successes. Before we start to figure out the best way to create goals, reflect on some of your thoughts and feelings about goals themselves:

- Make a list of goals you have set in the past (think about education, savings, projects, adventures, etc.)
- Examine each goal from the list above and mark it with an **S** for "succeeded;" **F** if you feel that you failed in achieving this goal; or **M** for "something in the middle between complete success or failure.
- How did you feel when you succeeded in attaining one of your goals?
- What did you learn from the goals you marked as "failures"? How did what you learned from them help you

or discourage you?

- What do you think about the ones you marked as in the middle between success and failure? Can you reframe them to look at what was successful in them? Can you take any lessons from the parts that felt less successful?
- What are your greatest successes? What makes them great?
- What will it feel like to "succeed" in your journey toward better health? What are you afraid "failure" might mean or say about you?

GOAL SETTING

Goal setting is imperative to achieving just about anything you wish for in life. Think of it in terms of a written agreement that you make with yourself to work toward a specific result. Establishing goals can help us to remain accountable to ourselves. I like to imagine these targets in two ways: continuous objectives and outcome objectives. Continuous objectives would encompass goals that require consistent attention over a long period of time. Examples include keeping daily food records, tracking intake in an app, eating three meals a day, or using measuring cups. They need to be meaningful to you and should be done on a regular basis. They become a normal daily practice and never end. Outcome objectives are specific long-term goals that you will meet by performing continuous objectives. In this case, outcomes are contingent on how consistent we are with carrying out the continuous goals. An example of an outcome goal would be to lose ten pounds or to reach a pre-determined goal weight. When you reach your goal, you may stop there. You do not have to continue losing weight if you are happy with your results. You must maintain carrying out the continuous goals, however, to prevent re-gaining the weight you just lost.

When you set your goals, try to be as specific as possible so they are easy to measure. SMART goals are Specific, Measurable, Achievable, Relevant, and Time-based.[24] A goal, for example, of initiating an exercise regimen would not be considered a SMART goal. It is too vague and does not help you adequately monitor your progress. A better goal in line with SMART goals would be: I will start walking for ten minutes two days a week starting the week of the tenth. It is an achievable goal that you can easily track.

I had a patient who identified her lunches during the workweek as something she would like to improve. For many years, her normal routine was to purchase lunch out Monday through Friday. Lunch could be anything from salad to fast food with fast food occurring most frequently. When I asked her what goal she would like to set she stated, "I would like to pack my

---

[24] "SMART Goals," Time Management, MindTools, n.d. https://www.mindtools.com/pages/article/smart-goals.htm.

lunch from home every day starting next week." My first thought was she wanted to go from packing lunch none of the time to doing it all the time. It seemed, to me, that she might be setting her goal too high and, therefore, possibly setting herself up for failure. Why did I think that way? Goal achievement is a slippery slope. It does not take much to *feel* like we have failed. When this happens, it is not uncommon for people to become despondent and use that as an excuse to abandon the goal completely. All she would have to do is miss making her lunch just ***one*** day that week and negative thoughts could potentially develop and threaten her plan. We discussed her goal and the rationale for a more realistic target with the option of changing it over time to reflect her confidence level in meeting her goal. She was agreeable and decided on brown-bagging her lunch two days a week.

I followed up with her. She was grateful for not bringing lunch from home every day. She said she realized that would have caused far more stress than she was ready to take on at that time. She was able to try it out while maintaining her other responsibilities which included making her children's lunches and taking them to their extra-curricular activities. This individual had not considered the logistics of her household in relation to her goal. As time went on, her husband and her children assumed more responsibilities which allowed her to focus more on meeting needs that were important to her.

Pay attention to your expectations. More is not always

better, especially early in the world of changing our behaviors. Start with small goals and build on them. This will give you a chance to acclimate to the changes you put into place and help you identify areas of your life that don't conform with your goals. Your odds of sticking with a behavior change increase significantly if it is meaningful to you and is compatible with your present lifestyle.

EXERCISE

As a registered dietitian, I cannot emphasize enough the importance of monitoring calorie control for weight reduction. You may wonder about the need for exercise. The real value of exercise in relation to weight lies in weight maintenance after weight loss. Using exercise alone without modifying our intake will make weight loss virtually impossible not to mention exhausting and frustrating! Below you will find some exercises performed at various intensities and the calories expended by a person who weighs 154 pounds when engaged in the exercise for sixty minutes. Keep in mind that calories burned per hour will be higher for people who weigh more than 154 pounds and lower for those who weigh less. A more extensive list, adapted from the Dietary Guidelines for Americans 2005, can be found in Appendix E at the back of the book.[25]

---

[25] "Calories/Hour Expended in Common Physical Activities," U.S. Department of Health and Human Services and U.S. Department of

Calories Burned in 60-minute activities[26]

Activity	154-pound person
Aerobics	480
Bicycling (<10 mph)	290
Running/jogging (5 mph)	590
Stretching	180
Walking (3.5 mph)	280
Weight Lifting(general light workout)	220

Calories in a single serving of snack foods[27]

Snack Food

Cookies, crème filled	2 cookies	140
Ice Cream	½ cup	150-210 (varies)
Peanuts	¼ cup	215

Agriculture. Dietary Guidelines for Americans, 2005. 6th Edition, Washington, DC: U.S. Government Printing Office, January 2005.

[26] Ibid.

[27] Giant. "Product Search." N.d. https://giantfood.com/product-search/.

Potato chips	1 oz. (10 chips)	150
Ritz® Crackers and cheese	5 crackers, 1 oz cheese	180

If we compare calories consumed to calories expended during *thirty* minutes of exercise in the above examples, we find that it's close to the same amount. If one of the biggest barriers to exercise is lack of time, then it hardly seems worthwhile to spend thirty minutes exercising to turn around and neutralize the deficit you just created by consuming ten potato chips or half a cup of ice cream. What if you eat more than ten chips or more than half a cup of ice cream which would not be difficult? Then the calories consumed increase. If you are trying to lose weight through exercise alone, you will have to increase the amount of exercise to sixty minutes to offset the snacking in the previous example. It is basic math, the more you eat the more exercise you require. It's not realistic to think we can exercise away all the calories we consume. I know I wouldn't want to try it!

Don't let the numbers discourage you. Having facts and information that we can use to make thoughtful choices is never a bad thing. I want to open your eyes to how easy it is to consume a considerable number of calories in a relatively small amount of food and how hard it is to remedy that through exercise. The other potential issue with exercise is that we tend to do less of it as we age. I always say to my clients, "At fifty, you are not doing what you did when you were twenty-five, and you most likely won't be as active at seventy as you are at fifty." It may not be practical to think we can control our weight through aggressive exercise especially if we try to sustain that level of activity as we get older. It is far more important that we do a moderate amount of exercise to preserve our muscle mass as we age intending to maintain our independence and quality of life. Exercise also plays an important role in helping us sustain any weight loss achieved through dietary modification.

If you are having difficulty initiating exercise, what can you do about it? Start with setting small exercise goals and work your way up from there. The message here is to gently persuade your mind to be at ease with changing your routine. If you attempt too much too quickly, you will most likely get backlash from your mind in the form of mental resistance. You will stop because it is telling you that it's "too hard" or "I don't have the time for this." Your mind is trying to keep you in that well-established territory that you are so accustomed to living in. From an evolutionary perspective, our minds are hardwired to go into safety mode when there is a threat of change. It wants to know, "How will this change affect me?" It cannot decipher if the change will produce good or bad results for us. Goal setting is a great way to slowly ease your mind out of its comfort zone. A perfectly adequate goal might be to go for a ten-minute walk two days a week. It seems silly because it's such a small amount of time, but it's ideal for facilitating change. Once you can wrap your mind around the idea of fitting exercise into your daily schedule, then you can consider increasing the frequency or duration of your walks until you reach your ultimate goal. This is how you create a new habit. Soon, exercising will be no different than brushing your teeth. You will do it because it's something that you value as an important part of your day.

The American College of Sports Medicine recommends that all adults do a minimum of 150 minutes of aerobic exercise a week. The recommendation for weight loss is between 200-300 minutes of physical activity a week. One hundred and fifty (150) minutes equates to thirty minutes five days each week and three hundred (300) minutes a week is sixty minutes five days each week.[28] Once you get used to doing the recommended amount then consider either increasing the frequency, duration, or intensity of the exercise to reap additional exercise benefits.

Get creative with your exercise routine. Your body needs to be continually challenged. I was used to walking my dog on a flat trail. Even though we would walk for one to two hours my

---

[28] U.S. Department of Health and Human Services. *Physical Activity Guidelines for Americans, 2nd edition.* (Washington, DC: U.S. Department of Health and Human Services, 2018), 8. https://health.gov/our-work/physical-activity/current-guidelines.

body got used to the routine. I was not seeing any improvement in my leg strength. I began walking with a friend who walked her dog on a path in local fields close to our homes. Once I started walking with her, I soon realized that it was more of a hike than a walk. I was continuously going up and down hills. I have been hiking now for about two years. My legs have become noticeably stronger and there is an obvious increase in my lung capacity. Changing my routine has improved my health. If you have the aerobic side of exercise down, then contemplate adding strength training to your regimen. Building muscle mass through light weightlifting will increase your metabolism and aid with calorie burning, therefore, making it easier to maintain a healthy weight. According to the Department of Health and Human Services[29], as little as 20-30 minutes of strength training 2-3 times a week can significantly improve muscle strength.

It is common to think that exercise will deplete your energy and make you even more tired than you already feel on a daily basis. Regular exercise, however, actually energizes you. Studies have demonstrated that exercise does wonders for our

---

[29] Mayo Clinic https://www.mayoclinic.org/healthy-lifestyle/fitness/in-depth/strength-training/art-20046670#:~:text=You%20can%20see%20significant%20improvement,Aerobic%20activity.

mental health and well-being.[30] Our bodies are designed to move. Unfortunately, that is often not emphasized enough when we are young. Being active on a regular basis is just one of those things that is hard to initiate, but once it becomes a part of your normal routine you will miss it if it doesn't get done. I have found that to be true for myself and I trust that you will feel the same way.

STRESS MANAGEMENT

Weight management, as we are learning, is multifactorial, and monitoring your food intake and exercise are only two parts of the equation. Stress is another major factor. Stress is categorized in two ways: acute or chronic. Acute stress is short-term occurring only for brief periods of time. Examples of short-term stress are being late for an important meeting, altercations, traffic jams, and deadlines. Chronic stress is long-term in nature and can last for months or even years. It may include chronic illnesses, job loss with the inability to pay the mortgage and other bills, an unsatisfactory marriage or relationship, a lengthy divorce, or the death of a loved one. Our minds and bodies can handle short-term stress and recovery happens relatively quickly.

---

[30] U.S. Department of Health and Human Services. *Physical Activity Guidelines for Americans, 2nd edition.* (Washington, DC: U.S. Department of Health and Human Services, 2018), 40. https://health.gov/our-work/physical-activity/current-guidelines.

Situations that keep us in a state of prolonged stress can have a negative impact on our health over time. In today's fast-paced world, many of us spend a significant amount of time in a state of chronic stress. Learning appropriate coping skills is imperative to negotiating the stress in our lives. While the bottom line of any diet is total calories consumed versus total calories expended, it is important to take inventory of everything that influences our actions if we wish to achieve long-term success. Bouts of stress are prompted by perceived threats in our environment. They induce the release of hormones to help us contend with the threat. This "fight or flight" response causes the brain to think it requires fuel to prepare for a scuffle, and we begin to crave sugar and fat in the form of "comfort foods". Stress drives some individuals to eat more and others to lose their appetites altogether until the stressful situation has passed.[31]

It should be noted that stress can impact our sleep and exercise patterns. When we are tired while trying to get through a difficult stressful time, our inhibitions are down, and we make poor food choices. This is also referred to as emotional eating. It

---

[31] "How Stress Can Make You Eat More – Or Not at All," Cleveland Clinic, last modified July 1, 2020, https://health.clevelandclinic.org/how-stress-can-make-you-eat-more-or-not-at-all/#:~:text=When%20you're%20feeling%20stressed,threat%20is%20causing%20the%20stress.

is usually mindless attempts to distract us from the pressures of our surroundings. Out of this maladaptive way of coping, we may create some bad habits that are hard to terminate after the stress is gone.

So, what can be done to manage our stress in the present moment and prevent undesirable patterns from developing? Start by maintaining as normal a routine as possible, adhering to eating, exercise, and sleep schedules. Just because there is tension in your life doesn't mean you can't go for your daily walk. In fact, physical activity may act as a form of relaxation or meditation and can be used to quiet your mind. This will help you sleep better and make better food choices. Making healthier food choices aids in sustaining emotional stability. Sugar and caffeine, especially in combination, are not very calming substances. Be sure to have healthy snacks available and be deliberate in choosing them. Everything is interconnected. Falling out of balance in any area has the potential to affect other areas.

Adopting and practicing stress management techniques on a regular basis will keep you prepared for the unexpected. We all know that stress frequently occurs unexpectedly. Guided meditation, yoga, deep breathing, engaging in hobbies, exercise, and spending time in the company of positive people are all activities that will have a calming effect while controlling your response to stress. I have a difficult time meditating. I can't seem to sit quietly for a long enough period to derive any benefit. I get frustrated with the process, which is the exact opposite of what I want. Therefore, I do not engage in meditation for my serenity. I much prefer to take long nature walks with my dog. It provides me with the necessary alone time to become calm. Find what works for you and set time aside to do it regularly. Always remember to "keep calm and carry on." I understand this is easier said than done.

SETTING GOALS WITH JANET

Picking up with her enthusiasm after her first two weeks of mindful eating and recording, it was time for Janet to set some goals. At first, Janet wanted to set a goal of losing 68 pounds in 6 months. "Janet, I love that you are excited and want to really go all in on your weight loss goals, but I want you to make goals that don't set you up for failure. Goals that are overly ambitious or that don't have a realistic chance of being attained can actually be de-motivating; we set a hard goal, don't make it, and then feel as if since we failed we shouldn't even bother. I want you to set goals that you can meet, and to allow meeting your goals to further motivate you."

We talked through the ideas of SMART goals, and the areas she might want to create goals in. We decided that Janet would set goals in three areas: weight loss, exercise, and mental health.

For her weight loss goal, Janet decided that she would aim

to lose a pound a week and shoot for an initial weight loss of ten percent of her present body weight (about 18-20 pounds). Although this wasn't as fast as she originally hoped, it's a specific, measurable goal that fits within realistic parameters given her life constraints and age. (And if she exceeded it each week, that would feel like a greater victory!)

To help her stay on track with her weight loss goal, we set an exercise goal. Janet doesn't love going to the gym, so she decided to set a goal to walk for forty-five minutes four times a week. Walking is something that she felt comfortable doing; it didn't need any special equipment, and she could do it alone or with a friend. "I think I'll find a special podcast that I only listen to when I'm walking--that way when I want to know what's happening next, I will know the only way to find out is to grab my walking shoes!"

Finally, Janet set a mental health goal. She decided that she would ask her best friend Lisa to walk with her one day a week to keep up her motivation and that she would reward herself for each week's measurable success by saving $5 toward getting a fancy massage. She also reached out to see what kind of support her doctor and therapist could give her for her journey.

We decided that Janet would try these three goals for a month, and then re-assess at the end of the month to see if the goals needed any tweaking, once she had some data to look at.

“Janet, those are some great goals. You’ll be able to measure them and see how much progress you make. Your goals will shift over time, but your relationship to creating good goals and celebrating your successes will be part of your life forever. I have a friend who says, ‘Practice makes permanent’ and I think it’s fantastic to think of the practice itself as being worth celebrating. You will be learning and growing on this path forever, and being happy about the process will help you have a positive experience.”

CHAPTER SIX: BEYOND THE NUMBERS

JANET'S JOURNEY CONTINUES

Janet was doing great! We met once a month for the next six months, and each time we met we compared the goals she had set with how the month had gone. In the first three months, Janet met her exercise goal of walking four times a week, and she was feeling very positive about her success. "I can't believe it! I grew up hating gym class, and going to the gym was even worse. But walking actually makes me feel better physically and mentally. If I skip a day, I find myself missing it and planning to make it up. I never thought I'd be here." Each month she took off her shoes and got on the scale--reluctantly. But after three months of losses exceeding her goals, she started to actually *look forward to getting on the scale*. After the first six months, Janet had upped her walking to five days a week, saved enough for her massage, and lost a total of *thirty-five pounds*, putting her more than halfway to her goal. At that visit, she did a little dance around my office.

"Robin! You've helped me so much! I never thought I could do this, but you made the steps make so much sense. My weight loss has been slow and steady. People keep telling me that I look great. Even if they don't say something about my weight (which is actually pretty nice, because I'm not a big fan of people commenting on other people's bodies), they say I look younger, or happier. And they're right! I feel younger, and I am really proud of myself which makes me happy!"

Things were going well for Janet, but she mentioned that she was going to a wedding in a couple of weeks, and she was having mixed feelings about it. "On the one hand, I'm excited because I will be able to wear a dress in a size I think I last wore in college. On the other hand, going will break my regular routine. I won't have my walking buddy, Lisa, I will have to travel, eat in restaurants, and there will be a wedding cake. What should I do?"

"Life is always going to interrupt, Janet. The thing to remember is that you are in control and you always have a choice. You can choose to walk by yourself, or on the treadmill at your hotel, you can choose meals in restaurants that you know meet your specific food goals. Don't be afraid to tell them that you have dietary needs and would prefer things like no dressing, no cooking in butter, and no sauce. You can request a take-out box at the start of the meal and put half of the portion right into the box before you even start. There are all sorts of ways that you can stay in control of what's going on. And don't forget--you're not always going to have a perfect week. Maybe you'll decide that you'd really like a glass of champagne to toast the happy couple, or that the wedding cake looks too good to pass up. You might add an extra day of walking to help make up for it or eat a big salad at lunch instead of a heavier meal, or you might know that the scale could go up a bit, but that you have the tools to bring things back into line after the interruption. As long as you remember that you are in charge of your choices rather than a victim of circumstance, you can deal with anything. You aren't dieting, you aren't using a quick fix. You are changing your life habits forever, and sometimes you will choose to splurge a little before going back to your regular, healthy habits."

Janet said, "I should set a SMART goal just about the wedding trip. That I will walk every day, and that I will choose one indulgence and really enjoy it."

At our next visit, a couple of weeks after the wedding, Janet stepped on the scale again. Her weight had dropped by three pounds, a pound less than she'd normally expect. I could see on her face that she wasn't delighted, but she said, "I managed to eat pretty well and keep up with my SMART goal about exercise. I would have liked to lose as much as I normally do in a month, but life interrupted. I'm glad I had that piece of cake. If I had been the only one not eating it, I would have felt really weird. And it was delicious."

I made sure that Janet knew that she'd done a great job. "I'll see you next month, Robin! I'm feeling really good about getting back to my regular routine!"

MOTIVATION

Janet was doing a great job staying motivated. Her initial impulse was to lose weight to be healthier, but as she moved along her weight loss journey, other factors started to motivate her, like feeling happier, being proud of her newfound ability to exercise, or fitting into a smaller dress size. Motivations can be small or big, external or internal, and they can (and should!) change during your own journey. I'd like to ask you to take some time to think about what you think about motivation:

- If you look back on your example goals from the last chapter, what were the things that kept you motivated to meet those goals? How did you save money, or get that job you wanted? How did you stick to your plans even when things were difficult?
- How do you feel about routine? Does it feel comfortable and make you feel more in control because you know what to expect, or does it feel confining? Make a list of all the positive and negative things you think about keeping a routine.
- How do you stay motivated when you are tired? When you are stressed or depressed? When you aren't getting the outside support you'd like? What are the things that make you feel more motivated? What discourages you?
- What has been the biggest stumbling block to your successful motivation in the past? Why do you think it has caused problems for you? What are some ways you can break that pattern? What kind of support do you need to break old habits? Who can you get that support from?

Yourself? Your spouse or partner? Your friends?

- What do you think motivates other people in your life? What can you learn from them (either good habits or things to avoid)?
- Do you believe that you have the power to meet your goals? Why or why not?
- What external things motivate you (such as numbers on the scale, smaller sizes, praise)? What internal things motivate you (such as pride in your accomplishments, happiness at improving your life, and the desire to be in control of your life)?
- What's the relationship between motivation and hope?

JANET RETURNS TO MY OFFICE

A month later, Janet came to our appointment. At this point, she'd been working on her weight loss journey for about eight months. She was more than halfway to making her final weight goal. She told me she'd kept up her walking routine, set a new goal for saving up money to get a massage as a treat for her walking buddy Lisa, and was excited to see where the scale said she was. She kicked off her sneakers and practically jumped onto the scale.

It read exactly the same number as it had a month ago. Janet stepped off and said, "That can't be right. Let me try again." She stepped back on again and let the numbers settle. I saw tears well up in her eyes. The number was the same again. "I've been so good. Why is this happening?"

"Janet, it's ok! Weight loss is a long journey, and people almost always hit a plateau somewhere along the way."

"What's a plateau? I can't believe this. I did everything I was supposed to. I feel like I'm being punished. Why should I even bother being so careful?"

I explained to Janet that a weight-loss plateau is a period of 'stalling' or even weight gain on our weight-loss journey. No healthy, sustainable weight loss journey is linear and the plateaus are important for long-term weight loss. "A plateau means that you have already had success in losing weight. You've lost pounds and moved toward your health goal. Congratulate yourself instead of feeling bad. A plateau is telling you that your body has gotten used to the place that you're in--the amount you're eating and the amount you're exercising. It's the body's way of telling you that it's time to make another change, and to set a new goal."

Janet said, "But I'm happy with my eating, and with my walking!"

"And you can remain happy with it if you want to stay where you are."

"But I want to reach my goal!!"

"To do that you're going to need to change something. You can lower your calories, or change your exercise. Now that you're used to walking so much, maybe you can consider switching it up. What if you traded one walking day for a yoga class or an exercise class at a gym? You're so much more confident than you used to be. I think you could face the gym now because you're much fitter, much slimmer, and much more confident. Maybe Lisa would take a class with you."

"Maybe what I should do is switch to a different program. One of those weight loss apps, or maybe I can get shots prescribed by my doctor."

SOME THOUGHTS ON QUICK FIXES: FAD DIETS, WEIGHT LOSS DRINKS, MIRACLE SHOTS

I would encourage you to speak with your physician to discuss medication and surgical options for weight loss. Gather some data so that you can make an informed decision about moving forward with your weight loss goals if you choose to take a different path. Remember, the choice of how you care for your body is yours and yours alone. My experience, however, is that a quick fix without behavior modification is a recipe for disappointment. Fad diets don't generally work. Establishing new habits that become part of a new way of living leads to much greater success than alluring fad diets. Rather than embracing a healthier lifestyle, they simply appeal to our desire to follow the path of least resistance—and we're learning how to work through that resistance! Let's explore this concept in relation to these trendy diets. People fall into the trap of believing fad diets are an easy and pain-free route to weight loss. This might be true if they worked over the long term, but, unfortunately, they can be difficult to sustain over time and weight regain is often the result. People find fad diets appealing because they frequently offer quick results and are easy to follow for a short time. Weight loss develops as if by magic, with relatively little effort on the part of the individual. More often than not, however, the weight loss is due to a decreased caloric intake, which is the ultimate goal of any diet plan. You can identify fad diets by their lack of balance and/or the elimination of major food groups. Cutting out whole grains, fruit, and low-fat dairy, for instance, means missing out on vital nutrients needed to maintain optimal health. The weight loss process is like a marathon. You win the race by being consistent over the long haul without doing anything radical.

Believe it or not, weight loss surgery requires one to follow a meal plan as well—a pretty strict meal plan at that. Guess what will happen if you don't follow the meal plan? You will likely regain lost weight. The difference here, though, is that your body has been altered through surgery and that cannot be changed. You may be at greater risk for many nutritional deficiencies after the surgery, even if you regain the weight. That may be a lifelong problem that your doctor could address with you.

The newest advancement in medication-driven weight loss is the use of GLP-I receptor agonists which slow the digestive process so that people feel full and consume less. According to the drugmaker's website, a 68-week medical study showed that taking the once-weekly injection helped people taking it to lose fifteen percent or more of their body weight while people taking the placebo lost two and a half percent[32].

"You've already lost that much weight on your own, Janet!"

Remember, you may lose weight while you are taking the medication, but what happens when you stop taking it? A good question for your doctor would be how long a person could stay on the medication and what are the long-term side effects of it. Again, if we have not made an effort to change our behavior and to make better choices, we will have difficulty maintaining any weight loss that we experienced while taking the medication. It might be worth it, in the long run, to invest the time now in making changes.

"All of those different alternatives may show you some quick gains, but nothing is going to replace you setting and meeting your own goals, and using tools that put you in control of your own choices. I know that facing a plateau is discouraging, but sticking with your big goals and adjusting your food and exercise goals to help you overcome this obstacle will be more

---

32 https://www.novomedlink.com/obesity/products/treatments/wegovy/efficacy-safety/clinical-trial-1-results.html

successful for the rest of your life, Janet."

The tears that had welled up in her eyes when she stepped on the scale fell down her cheeks. She was sad but also angry. "You don't know how this feels. You're thin and you've been thin all of your life!"

"I don't usually share this with my clients, but I have had my own challenges maintaining my usual weight. I'm not trying to say that I've faced the same situation that you are facing, but I do know how it feels to have to watch what I eat and how much I exercise. I have been doing those things all of my adult life. I'm finding as I age that what I was used to doing to maintain my usual weight isn't working as well as it once did. I've had to make changes to maintain my weight. Let me tell you my story."

MY WEIGHT LOSS STORY

We have examined some of the core beliefs that prevent people from making positive, long-term changes to their diet, sometimes before they even get started. Before we continue, I want to share my recent weight loss experience with you. My story demonstrates how our thinking can sabotage our efforts, even for a dietitian!

Maintaining my weight over the years has, for the most part, occurred in a relatively natural manner, much of which I attribute to my profession. I am not certain if it's my background in nutritional science or if food is just less appealing because I spend so much time talking about it. Something, however, has influenced me. As I've gotten older, my weight has become more difficult for me to manage. Being cognizant of what and how much I consume is more important now than previously. Becoming aware of my "food" thoughts has been one of the most valuable aspects of this journey. I would like to share some of my observations with you.

About a year ago, my weight reached an all-time high. I found myself just outside of a normal BMI for my height and weight. I had noticed that my weight was creeping up for some time, but the voice in my head kept telling me that "as long as I fit into my pants, I'm OK". We all know, however, that there is fitting into your pants comfortably and fitting into your pants like a sausage. I regrettably allowed myself to get to the uncomfortable sausage stage and was desperately trying to convince myself that this increased weight was not a problem and that I was in control. My normal lifestyle behaviors hadn't really changed. Then it occurred to me what might be causing my gradual increase.

What I failed to consider is that we start losing a small percentage of our lean muscle mass every year after age 30 (or 35) so our metabolism naturally slows down. Even though we are eating and exercising the same way we always did our bodies are changing and we start to gain weight. This is what caused my weight gain over a 10-year period of time. It came on slowly so it was easy to look the other way.

It would have been easy to let my ego step in and tell me that none of this was my fault, it was all just because I was aging. But the truth is, I know better. Years passing without aging isn't a possibility. I would have to face up to the fact that I would need to make adjustments to the way that I live to maintain my healthy weight.

To do this, though, I had to be willing to listen to my irrational self-talk. It was important for me to hear it and make the decision to hold myself accountable. In essence, I was lying to myself by saying everything was fine because I was still "able to fit into my pants." I knew that wasn't true. I acknowledged that if I continued to accept the lies that I was telling myself, I would never lose the weight. Ultimately, I wanted to lose the weight more than I wanted to continue with my present behavior. You will need to hear yourself and make a commitment to change the habits that need changing. Accept the fact that you may vacillate for a while until you are ready. Don't give up! Losing ten to fifteen pounds sounded like a reasonable place for me to start. I did what I am teaching you in this book. I selected a calorie level from the Meal Wheel. I got to work!

Appreciating the importance of being prepared, I took the time to plan out my daily meals and snacks to make it easier to adhere to my meal plan. I also vowed to start keeping a daily food journal. Vowing to start logging my food intake may have been a mistake as to vow is "to solemnly promise to do a specific thing",[33] but not necessarily doing it.

To be honest, I was initially resistant and did not start recording my food intake immediately. I can only speculate as to why. Possibly, I felt that I didn't have to keep records because I am schooled in nutrition. I "know what I am doing." Perhaps it was because I wasn't ready to face that writing my intake down "makes it real". Recording my intake means I actually consumed the food. If it is visibly transcribed on paper, then I'd have to address it. Whatever my reason, I was not ready. I had to discover for myself that I was never going to lose weight without taking the appropriate steps to make it happen. When I think back, what is comical to me, is that I am a registered dietitian. I am an expert in this field. Even so, I am human and not above getting caught in a mind trap, which is simply the way we react or cope with our experiences in life. There was an obvious level of resistance with which I was dealing, and I would have to find my own way of breaking through it. I was not prepared, in hindsight, to be fully candid with myself when I decided to make this commitment to lose weight. I wasn't willing to fully concede to a new modus operandi. Confronting the real issue at hand, and refusing to

---

[33] *Merriam-Webster Dictionary*, s.v. "vow," accessed Feb. 24, 2021. https://www.merriam-webster.com/dictionary/vow.

embrace change, would be my greatest challenge.

There were actions that I was already taking such as measuring out my food portions. I am proud to state I have been doing that faithfully every day for many years. I suggest you do the same. My boyfriend even measures out my food on the nights he cooks. Don't be afraid to lean on your family, friends, and your community for support as well.

It's wonderful that my boyfriend supports me in my choices, and helps me to stay on track with my goals. Because we are different people, with different goals, sometimes what works for one of us doesn't work for the other. I'm not a big snacker—I can go long periods of time without craving between-meal snacks. But sometimes when my boyfriend does the grocery shopping, he buys treats that I would normally pass by in the store. When they're right there on the counter (he loves to store them there instead of in the pantry, so they are easy for him to get to) I can't help taking a bite. I call this "drive-by snacking," when I just grab something on my way through the kitchen.

Like a lot of people, I sometimes snack when I am bored or distracted. When I'm sort of half-watching a television show in the evening, my mind can wander, and then my body wanders to the kitchen. I don't do this when I'm reading, or when I'm on the computer, so to keep my mindless snacking to a minimum, I limit the amount of time I watch TV—and try to only watch things I'm actually interested in, that keep my attention.

Another trigger for me that leads me right to a snack is stress. When I've had a hard day, I reach for something that I think will make me feel better, but when snacks add up to lots of unexpected calories, that momentary enjoyment can lead to longer-term regret.

Snacking isn't terrible—sometimes we all get hungry between meals (often when our meals aren't well-balanced) or after extra exertion (I like to give my dog a snack after we've gone on a good walk, and I sometimes need one, too). What doesn't support me in my weight loss (or maintenance) goals is when I'm not mindful about what I'm snacking on or why I'm snacking in the first place.

When it came to my own weight, I did not want to give credit to my habits for having a negative impact on my weight. In fact, I would often think to myself, "I don't eat that much. I'm not sure what caused the weight gain." Our habits, however, pose a substantial problem when it comes to monitoring caloric intake as they are difficult to account for especially if one is not tracking what they are eating. To compound matters, I found myself becoming frustrated because my weight wasn't changing. How could it? I wasn't even following my own advice. There were countless times when I would eat something that I didn't think I should be eating. Sometimes, I wasn't even hungry. My thoughts wavered, but they all led to the same conclusion—stop trying to change and go back to what was customary. I did begin to track my negative self-talk and was horrified by what I found. The following is a list of thoughts and feelings that surfaced in my mind at any given time during this process:

Oh, who cares?

This is too hard.

I'll start over tomorrow.

Who am I kidding?

You can't stick to anything.

You had that food that you weren't going to have—you blew it; may as well eat more.

This is a waste of time.

This is useless.

What am I doing this for-- I don't really look or feel too bad.

My clothes still fit

This doesn't work.

I had no choice but to pay attention to that last statement, "This doesn't work." After all the times that I had heard this from a patient and reminded them that putting in the effort the right way will always lead to success in the long run! I had to tell myself, "This **does** work, and you know it works. It's just never going to work the way you are trying to do it. It's time to change. Just surrender and do it the right way!" When I told myself to surrender and change, I felt lighter, as if a burden was lifted off my shoulders. There was a shift and I knew I was headed in the right direction. I downloaded the "My Fitness Pal" app and started tracking my intake. I even began pre-entering the foods I planned on eating the next day to ensure I would adhere to my meal plan.

What I am about to relate to you next may be difficult to hear and understand. I did not lose weight immediately. Three months passed before I started losing weight. *Three months!* I understand that everyone loses weight at a different rate, but the length of time it takes to see results is a key reason why people abandon their diets too soon. We want to see results in a short period of time. If we don't see at least some return on our investment in a week or two we convince ourselves that the effort is pointless and we stop. We develop a convenient reason to discontinue our dieting attempts while the real reason we stop is that we are not ready to change. I powered through those feelings because I know that the method I'm teaching you in this book works.

It took some time, but once I reached the "sweet spot" the weight came off relatively easily. I lost twelve pounds. That time interval can become a real mind game. I had to keep encouraging myself to "stick it out". I knew that weight loss doesn't always happen in our pre-conceived timeframe. I knew in my heart, though, that if I was consistent, patient, and persevered, it would work. I am convinced that this is the root cause of why people lose hope with weight loss. It doesn't happen fast enough. Disappointment sets in. People lose motivation. We come up with a litany of reasons to call it quits. I began to realize that I was eating better and becoming healthier. So, what else do I have but time? It took me ten years to gain the weight. It wasn't going to disappear overnight. I *chose* to give my diet a fair chance. It worked beautifully, just as I suspected it would.

I have kept the weight off for over one year now. I would like to lose another five to ten pounds, but I find myself in a similar place, mentally, to where I started. I can now understand what is involved in maintaining my present weight. Now I am able to spot the wrong reasoning I use to justify my dietary indiscretions. In other words, I have discovered what I am able to eat while still maintaining my new weight. I still measure all of my food out, but I have to admit that I slack off sometimes with My Fitness Pal. I accept that if I want to continue to lose weight, I must adhere more to my meal plan. It will take some time for me to surmount this next mental hurdle, but I know I can do it *if* I really want to.

Maybe that is why I had so much resistance at the beginning of my journey. I wasn't convinced that I really wanted or needed to lose the weight. Part of me wanted to have my cake and eat it too. I didn't believe I wanted to work that hard for something that came more easily for me in the past. Surprisingly, part of me was afraid I would not be successful in my attempt to lose the weight. My plan might not work *for me.* My body might respond differently to following a meal plan which may lead to failure. There go those pesky sabotaging thoughts again!

Sometimes we convince ourselves that the unknown will be worse than what is familiar. Is the risk worth the gain? Maybe we are just scared of what life could be like and settle for what life is because it's safe, easy, and convenient. We know where we are now, but we don't know where the road will take us in the future. If we don't try, though, we will never find out. Not taking the appropriate measures to obtain the desired outcome lies within the subconscious beliefs we hold. Start by following the Meal Wheel and then get to work on the real issues, the emotional blocks, that prevent you from losing weight.

My intention in revealing the previous information is to help you realize that there is a common thread to behavior change despite our different life situations and weight loss goals. Courage and dedication are required to obtain in life what you want. Individuals can spend their entire lives living in worry, fear, and doubt with thoughts about always falling short of attaining their goals. I am convinced that is why it takes me so long to get from point A to point B in almost everything I do in life. I don't want change to take as long for you. To go the distance, we must be willing and able to recognize, acknowledge, and ultimately change our beliefs. If you broaden your field of vision, life will unfold for you in unimaginable ways. Use your powers to obtain what you desire.

After hearing me tell her about my own experience, Janet felt a little better. "If even a professional has to watch what they eat and exercise to manage their weight, I guess I don't feel so bad. It makes sense that pretty much everyone has to put in some effort if they want results. So, can you help me decide on what changes I should make to break through the plateau and keep on track to meet my goal?"

We made some adjustments to her daily caloric intake using the formula and found her an hour-long exercise class that she would add once a week. She decided to buy some small weights to carry when she walked and armed with these new strategies, Janet headed home to recommit to her goals.

CHAPTER SEVEN: MAINTAINING, LIFELONG GOALS, SUCCESS

SO WHAT HAPPENS TO JANET?

You won't be surprised to know that Janet lost all the weight she planned to lose. She kept up with using the Meal Wheel. She adjusted her daily calories (knowing that the lower limit is 1200 calories, the minimum number to fuel a healthy body) and exercised every time she lost ten pounds, to minimize plateaus. She added a weekly exercise class with her friend Lisa, and then she added a second. By keeping her goals in mind and focusing on small SMART goals that built to her larger goal she was able to do what she never thought herself capable of when she first walked into my office. She started off at 185 pounds with a BMI of 30.8, and when she weighed in at my office on her "goal day" she was 147 pounds and a BMI of 24.5! Along the way, she learned that she could enjoy exercise, that she was stronger than she ever imagined (both physically and in terms of her will to achieve her goals), and that she really loved having knowledge and control of her relationship to food. She knew she could eat a piece of cake without ruining her entire diet, and that if she kept adding food to her diet her weight loss would bottom out, or worse yet--her weight would go back up!

"Well, I can't believe it! I did it! I am a success!"

"Of course, you are, Janet. I believed in you all along, and more importantly, you believed in yourself. Congratulations!" I gave her a small package.

"For me? Wow. Thank you!" She tore off the wrapping paper and revealed a journal. "This is so pretty. And it's blue, my favorite color. Thank you, Robin."

"It's for you to record your thoughts and feelings on this next step of your journey."

"Next step? Robin, I'm done! I met my goal."

"Janet, your relationship with food and movement will last a lifetime. You've made a fantastic start, losing the weight you wanted to lose. But you know from that journey that there are always bumps along the road. You will find new challenges as you move forward. You might backslide and gain weight again. You might find that your current exercise plan works great right now and then doesn't seem to do the trick anymore. You won't be losing weight toward a goal anymore, but you will be working to *maintain* your weight loss forever."

Like Janet, a lot of patients think that meeting the goal of weight loss means some sort of final success. That kind of thinking can be dangerous because people feel as if they can return gradually to old habits. Old habits bring back the same old weight problems. These are some ideas I always like to share:

- If you started this journey by telling yourself that you made the decision to permanently change certain behaviors, then once you get to the point of maintenance you will keep doing the new behavior. If you tell yourself that you just want to lose 20 pounds, once you get there your mind will think "What a relief, we are done" and that will make it hard to continue.

- People always ask me what to do after they lose weight. I tell them they need to keep doing what they have been doing otherwise the weight will go back up.
- Associating reaching your goal to a final destination is not a good idea. It implies that you can stop doing what you have been doing. The truth is it never stops, but it does get easier over time because it becomes your routine.
- There is always work involved, but what in life doesn't require work? Accepting that work is involved in creating what you want in life is the first step to getting what you want.
- It will also require conscious awareness to stay on course.
- You have seen Janet gradually learn how the Meal Wheel works, and how it corresponded directly to how successful she was. My hope for you is that by the time you get to maintenance, you have a good idea of what you need to keep doing to stay where you are.
- It's really all about self-esteem and self-worth. You have to believe that you are worth all the effort you will expend and that your health has value.

- If you have brown eyes, you don't spend a lot of time trying to make them blue, do you? (Okay, maybe you did when you were a kid, or maybe you have blue contact lenses). You have accepted that your eyes are your eyes. The same is true of your relationship with food. Sure, some people you know are rail thin and eat piles of pasta for every meal. That is them. You can't compare yourself to others, and you can't lament that your body system works differently than theirs. That would be like complaining that your eyes are brown.
- Life requires that you participate--in whatever comes up. No one's life is without challenge, but you can't fold up and stop trying when things get hard.

When my reason for giving her the journal started to sink in, Janet said, "When I hit that first big plateau, you told me about your own weight loss journey. I know that you've had to maintain that weight loss. What are some of the things you've done to do that?"

"I've followed the exact same rules as you. I record my food and measure what I eat. I make sure to maintain my exercise regimen. Weight loss isn't the only place in my life where I have faced difficulties or used these ideas to help myself. I try to be conscious of my emotional state, and to cultivate emotional awareness."

EMOTIONAL AWARENESS

Simply hoping that something good will happen to us is not enough. Life requires faith combined with action. You will need to have a clear vision of what you want to accomplish as well as the resolve to stay focused on the outcome. Taking the time to understand the driving forces behind your actions will help you with your long-term goals. Identifying which emotion that I am feeling has been a challenge for me. Accurately identifying your emotions is important as it determines how you interpret your life experiences. Your reactions and the decisions you make are based on your experiential evaluations. Learning to function at an emotionally positive level will keep you more in tune with the natural flow of life. It is in this flow where big changes occur. Being self-aware provides the opportunity to be with our authentic selves.

A great deal of research has been conducted on measuring the positive and negative frequencies of emotions. Everything in the universe has energy including your body, your thoughts, and your feelings. According to Sabrina Reber, author of *Raise Your Vibration*, "Distorted beliefs, fear, anger, resentment, blame, guilt, jealousy, judgement, shame, addiction, unforgiveness, conditional love, lack of self-worth, greed, separation consciousness, and poor health keep you in very dense, low vibrating energy."[34] When we operate in a sub-optimal inner state, we feel heavy, repressed and closed off to the world around us. Even those words "sound" burdensome. Our vibrational frequency then, at any point in time, creates the basis on which we formulate our thoughts. If we *allow* lower-level emotions to be predominant, then there is a strong potential for them to have a detrimental influence on our lives. To attract and obtain what we want, we must modify our thoughts and behaviors and accept and experience higher positive emotions.

The image that comes to mind when I think of positive and negative emotions is balloons tethered to weights. Like a balloon, we can go up and down. In my mind, the balloon is representative of higher positive emotions. It is the place where we have the most potential to grow and advance. It is where we feel good and are open to making positive changes in our lives. The weights, on the other hand, represent the opposite lower, negatively charged emotions that tend to pull us down and impede our ability to rise to a higher state. They don't feel good and they keep us from experiencing the many wonderful aspects of life. The rope that connects the two is our in-between emotions. Once we anchor ourselves in a low-level place, it becomes very difficult to break

---

[34] Sabrina Reber. *Raise Your Vibration.* (North Charleston, SC: CreateSpace Independent Publishing Platform, 2013). 4.

free. If we can chip away even the smallest pieces of the weights we carry, we begin to move in the right direction.

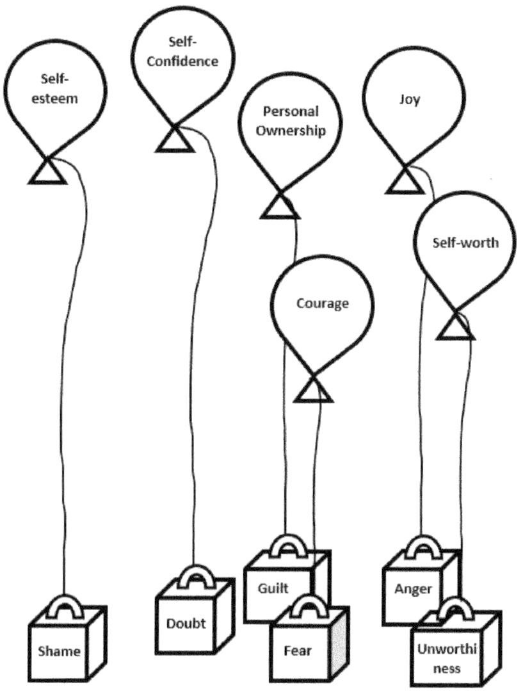

It wasn't until I was able to connect an appropriate emotion to my reactions to outside stimuli that everything started to improve for me. Shame, for instance, was not a feeling that I readily identified with until it was pointed out to me by my energy healer.

I had a neighbor, who I considered a friend, come over to my house one day while I was weeding. She insulted my property. Her statements felt like an unsolicited attack. Of course, I took it personally and became infuriated. It wasn't until I shared this story with my energy healer that I was able to make a connection to what was taking place emotionally inside of me. My healer asked me, "What were you feeling?" I responded, "Angry." She said, "No, that is not it. What were you feeling?" Again, I replied, "Really angry." She went on to explain that my neighbor triggered the emotion of shame, not anger, which I probably experienced some time in childhood. This experience must have made me remember someone saying something or treating me in a way that caused me to feel inadequate and it shifted me into a well-established *story about myself.* I have often found it hard to identify what I am feeling because my triggers always appear to come from *outside of me*. I automatically direct anger at the other person. I had to learn what was taking place *inside of me* that was causing the emotion. This pervasive feeling of shame made me angry that day.

My feelings went much deeper than anger. It never occurred to me that my self-esteem could be impaired—that it was about me. I had constructed so many walls trying to protect some false sense of self that I could not understand what it was that I was doing or feeling. To me, anger is protective. I could defend myself with anger, but shame meant that something was fundamentally wrong with me. Possibly, I unconsciously built walls to avoid looking objectively at the shame. Anger was the perfect cover-up. It wasn't until recently that I began to recognize that the shame I was experiencing originated from a self-created belief system of not being good enough. I fabricated this way of thinking based on my many life experiences. I would have to work on changing my beliefs if I wanted to break this cycle. I felt a great relief to finally make the association of my role in my emotional reactions.

Essentially, what we need to recognize and take responsibility for, in any given moment, are the feelings that we are experiencing within us. My neighbor had her own reasons for stating what she said. I will never know what gave rise to her remarks. Regrettably, I jumped into that comfortable state of projection and became angry *with this individual*. My feelings, though, were providing me with an opportunity to learn something about *myself*, not about the other person. Our reactions are rarely about the person we are in conflict with but rather are created out of our own beliefs. It turned out to be a wonderful learning lesson for me for which I am grateful.

Make no mistake, I do not condone people being cruel. I was within my rights to feel hurt, angry, and betrayed by my neighbor's words. I remained, however, in this angry state for far too long afterward. It is easy to be seduced by negative thoughts when they are triggered. I wallowed in my own self-pity after that incident. I gave all my power to that other individual.

I say, no more! Seek out resources around you that can help you find viable solutions to your emotional barriers. You don't have to do this alone. In fact, I am not sure I would have been able to make these connections without the assistance of a dear therapist and my energy healer. Pinpoint your feelings, own them and then let go. This will improve your emotional state and allow energy to flow.

Being hung up on the minutiae of day-to-day life obstructs the entire process. If you are angry with someone, your energy level will match that feeling. If you are joyful, you will get more experiences that match that energy. Have you ever noticed that when you are upset things seem to keep going wrong? Or, when you are feeling in sync with the world around you, life goes more smoothly, and wonderful things happen? Keep your morale up, and do whatever is needed to keep functioning at a higher frequency. Then, you can direct your energy toward the things that are really important to you. This makes life so much easier.

Fear is another low-grade emotion that I am all too familiar with. Fear can paralyze. I am aware that I must manage mine more constructively, but whatever the circumstances I usually remain in it for far too long. What gets me past my fear? Facing it. For me, the dread of stagnation eventually overrides the fear of change. When I get tired enough of being frightened, I force myself to "rise up". I move up to a place of courage. I manage to get things done despite my fears. Trust me when I tell you that you will know when it's time to "rise up". This process requires you to really listen to yourself. I begin to alter my conduct when I can't bear to hear another complaint or worry come out of my mouth. I am simply drained when in a prolonged state of inactivity. When this occurs, I slowly start to face issues directly. For example, I will remain in a job long after I should because I am afraid to take a chance at a new job. It is so much easier to let inertia win. Most of my career changes came about because a more appealing opportunity became available rather than me seeking out a new position even though I may have wanted to find a better job. Through good discernment, however, I have been able to spot viable new opportunities and take them when they appear. This ability has kept me moving in the right direction. If you can get yourself to move up the balloon string, then you are on course.

I understand that it is now in my best interest to identify early what I am afraid of or ashamed of and find a way to change these feelings in order to regain equilibrium. When I want to rise above a negative vibrational frequency, I have to first gain clarity about my present state of mind [what am I *really* feeling?]. Then, gather up the courage and determination to make pertinent adjustments. Finally, I take the necessary action to improve my place. Remember, change ultimately requires action.

This book is a perfect example. I have wanted to complete this book for several years. I tried to remain inspired, but I continuously battled feelings of self-doubt and unworthiness when it came to completing this project. I found myself asking, "Who are you to write a book or want a different life?" or "How in the world are you going to accomplish this enormous endeavor? You can't do this." Writing a book is hard enough. Confronting the constant negativity of my unspoken thoughts was an entirely different job. It has been a long and arduous process, but I am glad I pushed myself out of my comfort zone.

What did I learn about myself during this undertaking? I learned that indifference has played a big role in the timeline of this activity and that maybe this is another form of fear that has kept me stagnated. Trying to stay motivated to complete this book has really tested my abilities to persevere especially considering I had no way of knowing if anyone else besides my editors would ever read it! My cynical inner voice had to change as well. In the beginning, I kept saying, "But, I am not a writer." How was I going to write a book if I kept reinforcing the belief that "I was not a writer?" Then I heard the saying that "books aren't written, they are rewritten." Those words were very encouraging. It was comforting to know that I didn't have to get it right on the first attempt. I was not alone. I could consult people who are writing experts. Together we could create a readable product. This positive conclusion convinced me to keep trying. What internally is blocking your path to success?

Some questions for you to consider at this point:

- What does success mean to you? Do you see it as a single occurrence of meeting a goal, or as an ongoing experience?
- What are the things about yourself that you accept the

most?

- What is your relationship with shame? Where does it come from in your life? What are the physical feelings of shame? What are the emotional ones?
- Where do you fall in the weight (negative feelings) versus balloon (positive feelings) scenario? What are some actions that you can take to begin your ascent to a better feeling place? What are some of the things you are saying to yourself that are literally weighing you down
- What are you afraid of? How will you move past your fear?

THE BUCKET LISTS

What do you want to do before you leave this Earth? Bucket lists are experiences or achievements that an individual aspires to accomplish during their lifetime. They are self-created and hold meaning only for the individual. The activities on a bucket list are considered exciting and challenging and we look forward to someday participating in them. We have complete control over what we place on the list. We make a *conscious* decision to choose them.

There are many circumstances in life over which we do not outwardly appear to have control. Some of these experiences we would rather avoid. I consider the situations in life that seem to be out of our control as our subconscious bucket list. It's the bucket list the universe has planned for us based on the contract we make before we are born. I believe our souls come here to gain knowledge acquired through experience. The encounters that we have allow us to learn and evolve if we are open to them. This bucket list is different as we do not knowingly choose the experiences on the list and yet we are actively creating them every day. Our thoughts and beliefs bring these experiences into our reality. The items on this list are often difficult to deal with and they provoke uncomfortable feelings. Facing these life challenges and conquering them is essential for emotional and spiritual growth. Our lessons can come from many different life experiences such as addictions, divorces, anxiety, and the death of a loved one. Life is not trying to beat us down when we face these types of adversities. Life wants you to find solutions to your problems. You create better ways to cope. That is what makes you strong. Our outcomes are dictated by our ability to judge well and how we handle difficulty. There are many directions we can take and they may lead to different outcomes. This could be considered a field of choices or possibilities. We can either learn our lessons or not. One thing is for certain; our lessons will keep appearing in our lives over and over if we continue to deny our reality. The choice is ours.

It is common to struggle with the subconscious bucket list because the situations we find ourselves in may be painful and cause suffering. They trigger the emotions and beliefs that we must transform in order to grow. This reminds me of the phrase "Life is like a game". We must confront this subconscious bucket list. Otherwise, we risk remaining in a permanent state of inaction. This is a healing journey. It is all about learning how to play the game.

This way of thinking has helped me deal with the vicissitudes of life. It puts me in the driver's seat rather than allowing me to believe that I am powerless to change my circumstances. It provides me with the opportunity to a be player rather than a spectator. I have spent far too much time on the sidelines mainly because I was too afraid or too unwilling to participate. It doesn't mean, though, that I didn't want to try, but rather I would not allow myself to be vulnerable. We are always in the process of creating our paths in life either passively or actively. It is in our best interest to face what life presents. I like to think of it as a cosmic to-do list. Framing it his way makes me less resentful for the experience, and more willing to try to succeed in dealing with a problem. I prefer to make my own decisions rather than have someone else make them for me.

As the main character of my game, I find myself hunting for clues to determine my next move. Signs almost always arrive from my surroundings. I love it when they resonate with me. My inner guidance system interprets these messages as either something helpful or a hindrance. I make decisions based on my internal feelings or intuition. We must learn to trust those feelings.

CHAPTER EIGHT: HOW THE LESSONS WE LEARN IN ONE PART OF OUR LIVES HELP US WITH THE OTHERS

One of the happy/sad parts of my work is that when people succeed at setting and achieving their weight loss goals (happy!) I often lose touch with them (sad!). I've taught them what they need to know in order to take control of their relationship with food and movement, and they will take that knowledge with them and work to maintain what they have accomplished.

Another of the happy/sad parts of my job is when I hear from a former client because they've lost their way and gained back some, all, or more of the weight--I'm pleased that I get to reconnect with them, but sorry that they are unhappy with their weight and feeling defeated. Here's the truth: it happens. There's no shame in backsliding, and the same tools that you used to succeed in your original weight loss are there to support you in getting back on track.

JANET COMES BACK

About a year after I last saw Janet, I saw her name come back up on my appointment schedule. I was pretty sure I knew what she was going to tell me.

"Oh, Robin! I'm so embarrassed to be back here! I've

gained back 12 pounds, none of my clothes fit, and I can't stand to look at myself in the mirror! I'm a complete failure. It's been three months, and every time I thought about reaching out for help, I felt sick. I thought you'd be so disappointed in me."

"Janet! It's ok. I'm not disappointed in you--it's not my job to judge you. And more importantly than that, you shouldn't care about how I feel. You should care about how you feel. You clearly don't feel good about gaining back some of the weight, but you have already taken steps to take control again. What made you finally decide to come back to see me?"

"I thought each month that the weight was a fluke and that it would stabilize soon. I was ashamed to need help, so I waited and convinced myself that it would be ok. But finally, I realized that it wasn't getting better, it was getting worse. I wanted to get help from you because this was the one thing I've done that I felt successful about!"

"I'm glad you came back to see me. I am always here to support you. What do you think should be our first step?"

As we talked, I asked Janet lots of questions--that led her back to The Meal Wheel. She'd been slipping in a lot of small ways--¾ of a cup of ice cream instead of ½, measuring a serving of rice by eyeballing it rather than using a measuring cup, skipping a workout here and a walk there. Every time I asked a question like, "How about trying a food journal for a few days to see how things are going there" or "What's your calorie target right now?" I could see in her eyes that all she needed was a little nudge back to the principles that we'd established in our first few meetings. All through the conversation, she remembered that she really *did* know what to do, and that she really *was* able to do it. As she got up to leave, she stopped and asked me, "Robin, did you ever find that making a change like this in your life was so hard that you felt like you needed more than just the rules to depend on? I mean, when you were losing weight, or trying out some other new skill in your life, did you want emotional or, I don't know, spiritual help with all of this?"

I had to give it to Janet, she'd honed in on something that I think many approaches to weight loss just don't give much time or attention to. We all have a desire for support and guidance, and although the Meal Wheel is exactly the tool you need to help you with the nuts and bolts of weight loss, I want to make sure not to neglect the other parts of you. My own experiences with growth and change in my life have provided me with a model for how to work for balance in my own life, and I hope that by sharing them I can help you, too.

But before we talk about that, I have some questions for you to consider:

- Where have you felt the most out of place in life? Where do you feel the most comfortable/authentic?
- Do you identify as religious or spiritual, (or both, or

neither?)? How has your spiritual side helped you with problems in the past? Or, why does a spiritual life not work for you?

- How has the family you came from impacted your spiritual side in positive or negative ways?
- When you fail at something, do you assign blame or responsibility? What comes after assigning that?
- What are you hanging on to? Is it time to let go?

FOOD FOR THOUGHT

There are components contributing to our well-being that extend beyond our physical bodies. The outside world is objective in nature in that we can attempt to explain our experiences using our five basic senses; touch, sight, hearing, smell, and taste. Our inner worlds of emotion and spirituality, however, are considered subjective and more difficult to describe due to their lack of a tangible form.

My struggles with the emotional and spiritual side of human existence have been ongoing since my youth. Difficult to articulate, I often felt out of place in day-to-day life. Even as a child, I sensed that there was a grander meaning than what I was experiencing in my immediate external world. Accomplishments were too frequently followed by inexplicable feelings of disappointment. Sometimes I didn't even want to try to excel simply due to a gnawing fear of disappointment and failure that followed me around. I had a very hard time comprehending why feelings of fulfillment and joy were eluding me.

Dreams of becoming an artist were dismissed as I was told that artists are eccentric and that artistic creation is only worth something after the artist is dead. I was told that I would never be able to support myself financially as an artist. A vivid memory from my childhood was when my father said to me, "Blend in Robin. Conform. Why would you want to be different and stand out?" I have carried this with me all of these years. It was perplexing to me, even as young as I was, that my father said this to me. All I heard was that I could not become who I wanted. Rather, I had to become who my family or society thought I should become. That was the start of my limited belief system based on what I was told by those surrounding me. I learned not to trust my inner self. Unintentionally, I allowed those words and the beliefs I constructed around them to affect the decisions I have made throughout my life.

Balancing out the negative with the positive is helpful when I am trying to sort through my feelings about the past. It is so much easier to recall the statements or actions that hurt me, but my experiences really have been a healthy combination of both "good and bad". My mother has told me about an interaction that she witnessed between me when I was five, and a ten-year-old neighbor girl. Apparently, I dressed myself in a red, white, and blue top, a paisley skirt, high white boots, and a broken headband. I proceeded to play with the other kids in the neighborhood. Yes, my mother let me go out dressed like that. This neighbor girl said to me, "That is the ugliest outfit I have ever seen." In turn, I said, "I don't care, I like it" and I walked away. I love that story because that was me being unapologetically me and nobody was going to change my thoughts. My mother was more comfortable allowing me to be the creative dreamer who was a little different from the other children. I danced to the beat of my own drum. My father, on the other hand, was more analytical and reality-based. He had trouble relating to a child with such a different outlook. He felt safe following social norms and not drawing attention to himself. All the messages that I received from the people in my life have left me confused in my adulthood as to what my actual path should be. Living with a subtle, yet chronic, underlying current that I am not living up to my fullest potential I realize it's time to make a change. I am in the process of finding my way back to that brave little girl. I am trying to find my own personal way.

Cultures indoctrinate their youth with narratives of how life works based on what they were historically taught by their ancestors. Seeds of beliefs may be planted that may not support the young person's higher purpose. Children are meant to shine, but grown-ups inadvertently take away their luster by instilling their own opinions into the youth. Adult communication can squash the aspirations of children and set them on a course in life that may not have been of their own choice only to find out later that it does not resonate with them. While this downloading of beliefs is occurring, we start to build the proverbial walls around our hearts. We become less open to the possibilities of our lives and underestimate our capabilities. The adult, undoubtedly, has good intentions and is trying to protect the child from disappointment, failure, and regret, but these exchanges turn into what I view as an assemblage of internal knots that are formed in the child to protect his/her self. We store these interactions somewhere inside our minds. Age-appropriate defense mechanisms are constructed to shelter us from the pain caused by these experiences. Sadly, we may bring these defenses into our adulthood where they no longer serve us, but rather hinder our progress. The key is to recognize and untie these knots or beliefs in adulthood if we want to appreciate the true joy of living. The feelings that surface when we are triggered are the first signal that something needs to be addressed within us. Explore the knots that you have tied for yourself. Where did they originate? What were some of the mistaken beliefs you created as a child that you might still be carrying with you? What will it take to untie them?

I will do my best to relate to you parts of my life story which I have come to accept as the untying of my knots—my path to emotional and spiritual awakening. The experiences I have had while unique to me, are in a broader sense, probably quite common. I now do not label them as good or bad. In fact, I feel that the purpose of the encounters with our families and with other individuals throughout our lives is to offer us enough contrasts to our own inner beliefs so as to wake us to our true selves and to provide us with the courage to live in accordance with our beliefs. Relationships are tools to be used in our emotional and spiritual maturation process—try to observe them in that context. This isn't to say downplay how important other people are in our lives, but rather to remind you that your relationship with yourself is the most important one that you will ever have. I hope that sharing this information serves you well on your journey. I invite you to take my examples and apply them to your own situation. You will have two tasks to work on simultaneously: weight loss and emotional self-discovery. Be excited to see where this takes you!

The first section of this book explains the Meal Wheel and the nutritional information that you need to get started with your weight loss. In this last section, I introduce you to aspects of eating that are more subtle and abstract in nature. It is information that I continue to study and practice. Consider this section food for thought. Perhaps you will not do anything with the information I provide here. That is fine. Something that I present, however, may resonate with you and could be the beginning of a whole new way of thinking about food and how you approach your life.

You may think the hardest part of following a healthy diet and trying to lose weight is the food aspect of the diet. You may be concerned that you will struggle with smaller portions or resent not being able to eat the foods you enjoy. While these are all valid feelings, and I talked about how to manage them briefly in the previous section, it's been my experience that the most difficult part of dieting and losing weight is trying to understand the thoughts or feelings that drive your *behavior* of eating. If it was just about the food, you would not have a problem following the Meal Wheel, or any other diet, and reaching success. The bigger issue is that we often take comfort in means outside of ourselves, such as food, to weather more challenging aspects of our lives. Emotions such as shame, guilt, fear, doubt, or unworthiness are often lurking in our subconscious. We may repeatedly use external ways to avoid internal pain and angst. Food can be a great distraction from our emotional world helping to mask the uneasiness of confusing feelings.

People self-soothe all the time in a variety of different ways. For some it may be drinking, taking drugs, gambling, shopping, or any other number of activities that help to divert our minds from the discomfort of our reality. Others turn to food. The act of eating something we enjoy can elicit a happy or joyful response in our body and temporarily lift us up and improve our mood. Your mind, however, is making it appear as if the food is causing you to feel better and that feeling convinces you to eat more. What other ways can you get that sensation or have that need met that doesn't involve food? In order to change our relationship with food, I propose that we contemplate doing some work from the inside out and release these trapped emotions to gain a different perspective.

The first step is becoming aware of some of the "doctrines" you have constructed around food, your weight, and your ability to produce the changes necessary to achieve your desired outcomes. A commonly held notion that has been frequently communicated to me by my patients is "I love food!" I say no: you love your family, your kids, and your dog, but not food. Is it possible that you are confusing the satisfaction derived from consuming food with adoration for the food itself? Is it the culture we have created around food that you enjoy? Socializing with friends and family around a good meal can be a very pleasurable experience. While I do think some individuals may enjoy food chemistry and the experience of cooking and tasting food, I commonly ask those patients to think about what is their actual investment in food. What would happen if you separated the act of eating from the act of socializing? Would you no longer enjoy the company of your friends and family? Would the food no longer provide the same level of gratification? Or, would you find different value in each experience that you didn't previously realize?

Other patients have shared memories from their childhood that revolve around the concept of deprivation. I've heard stories where food was withheld from the individual while their siblings were allowed second helpings. Furthermore, some were restricted from going into the refrigerator to get food. Some refrigerators were even locked! The response to these childhood experiences has left a subconscious decision to never again go without food. I have been told by many that they vowed, "When I get older, I am going to eat whatever I want. Nobody is ever going to tell me that I can't have something I want again." Connecting the association between a childhood experience and your present views about food is important. Certain situations may transport us back to childhood where we felt helpless. Remind yourself that you are no longer that child and will never be in that situation again. Take it one step further and ask yourself if that way of thinking is presently supporting you.

That's not to say that all childhood memories of food are negative. Some recollections have very positive associations attached to them such as grandma's homemade pasta and marinara sauce or being offered goodies as an expression of love. My grandmother always used to ask me, "Do you want a cookie? Can I get you something to eat? Are you hungry?" "*Mangia mio figlio*", ("eat my child" in Italian), were loving words that were spoken to me regularly. I used to eat what she proffered because I didn't want to hurt her feelings. Guilt is a significant emotion that we all experience. I experience a lot of guilt when I feel like I am not doing something that someone else wants me to do—that's probably why I ate what my grandmother offered. At some point, however, I learned to say no because I simply wasn't hungry. Being a "yes" person and wanting to please others had the potential to create a real problem for me. Unfortunately, if we don't identify and address the real issue at hand, that internal dialogue we have running in our minds will inhibit us from making headway in our effort to lose weight.

Another misconception is that having a different body will provide you with a better life. Do not look to your body to bring you happiness that it can't deliver. It is just a mass of cells. Your mind will have you believing your body is too big or too small or not the right shape for you to be happy. You have the power to change your thoughts. Don't give your power away to your body. It is not your body that is causing your suffering. Rather, the thoughts that you have attached to your body are causing your suffering. Your body can't do anything without your mind directing it. Learn to master your thoughts about your body and your attitudes and feelings about your physical appearance will all change.

Finally, is there a fear you hold that may accompany the thought of weight loss or of modifying your lifestyle? It is normal to be comfortable with the status quo and not want to change. Fear is usually the driving force behind change inertia, and it is important to recognize your self-generated fears. Let's consider what fear of weight loss or a change of diet might look like. Most of us are used to our daily routines. We favor our present way of living, even if it's not in our best interests. We even establish a hierarchy of our habits. Even though we maintain that we want to lose weight, we sometimes, unknowingly, place our eating habits above the desire to lose weight because we derive immediate relief or pleasure from food. Change can also be scary because we know what we've got, but we don't know what is going to come with change. What makes altering our relationship with food even more challenging, is that we are dealing with concepts that may be contradictory. We don't even notice the opposing thoughts. If we remain in this conflicting emotional state, we will most likely remain in the same physical place.

There are probably numerous ways we internally fight with ourselves every day. Examining a few examples of perceived positive and negative outcomes of weight loss may make you more mindful of your own dichotomous way of thinking. Write down everything that floats through your consciousness, as it will direct you on what to focus on later. Create two lists-- positive and negative. The positive outcomes list will describe desirable and exciting ideas you perceive experiencing after losing weight. The negative outcomes list will conjure up the more frightening concepts that may come from your current views about weight loss. The lists may contain competing inclinations. These contrary forces inside us make the undertaking of weight loss stressful and difficult. The following table presents some of the paradoxical thoughts and feelings that may reside inside the subconscious mind that need to be confronted so we can accomplish our goals and live the life we dream.[35]

Let's start with a checklist of ideas that I generated based on feelings I have identified about advancing my career. From there, we can analyze the potential pros and cons of losing weight. I anticipate that this exercise will reveal a common theme.

Positive Outcomes	**Negative Outcomes**
Seen by others as the expert	Seen by others as the expert
More recognition	More recognition
More responsibility	More responsibility
New and exciting job opportunities	New and exciting job opportunities
More earning potential	More earning potential

The positive outcomes list contains the points that I believe most people are looking for as their careers mature over time. As I contemplate what the future of my profession might resemble, I become apprehensive over the idea of not being capable of handling the responsibility or recognition of moving up the ladder

---

[35] Dr. Gail Saltz. "Conquer your fears about losing excess weight," *The Today Show*, June 28, 2007, https://www.today.com/health/conquer-your-fears-about-losing-excess-weight-wbna19488269.

in my chosen occupation. While being considered "the expert" in my specific discipline is an honor, it can be intimidating at the same time regardless of my educational background or extensive work experience. Initiating something new can be thrilling, but the uncertainty of uncharted waters is also unnerving. Venturing into the unknown is a bit like moving through the dark. What would a new job entail? Would I be able to live up to the expectations of a new role? Would I succeed? My controlling side always wants to know exactly how everything will develop, but that is not realistic.

The position I hold at my present place of employment came about very quickly. I had to decide to accept the job with very little time to think about all the aspects of the new position. I went through various emotions at that time. I distinctly recall worrying about whether I could actually perform the job. The responsibility of this new position felt unsettling. All of these thoughts and beliefs emerged when this opportunity was presented. What's interesting is that I was already doing the job! The woman who previously held the position had me tracking the data and running all the reports for the department even though she was ultimately responsible for the overall performance of the center. I had all the tools that I needed to be successful. Yet, I was struggling with the confidence to take on the new title, to accept more authority, and to work autonomously. These doubting feelings are nothing new to me. I have had to work consistently on altering the beliefs I have about my abilities and my self-worth which were likely conceived in my youth. If I allowed myself to dwell in that negative inner dialogue, I would never have taken the chance. I would never have progressed in my career. Fortunately, I didn't have much time to think about the new position. The quickness of the decision worked out to my benefit. I am also more aware of how I sabotage myself with my thinking. I continuously work on identifying and changing my negative thoughts and beliefs with the intention of furthering my career. Is it possible that you are wrestling with adversarial thoughts about weight loss? Let's investigate what might surface in terms of one's weight.

Positive Outcomes	**Negative Outcomes**
Seen by others as more attractive	Seen by others as more attractive
More attention	More attention
More career opportunities	More career opportunities
More social possibilities	More social possibilities

Again, almost any outcome can elicit both positive and negative thoughts or feelings. We may desire to become more attractive and receive more attention, but these desires can be very threatening if our belief system doesn't match up with our aspirations. Considering how we will navigate new and different situations can give rise to unintended anxiety. More opportunities in life sounds fantastic, but an unconscious concern might be that you will not be able to manage new opportunities that come your way. Changing the outside doesn't change the beliefs we hold on the inside. We attract what supports our belief system. We can't tolerate positive thoughts and negative thoughts taking place at the same time. Negative thoughts are pulling us in one direction and positive thoughts in the other direction. We get stuck somewhere in the middle. It is this discord in our subconscious that keeps us from advancing toward our goals. I do not mean to imply that we can make our negative thoughts go away completely. If we acknowledge them, however, and allow them just a small space within us, the grip they have on us will loosen and they will be less likely to hold us back.

It is possible that we have been using our excess body weight as an excuse over the years for not achieving what we want—relationships, careers, happiness, or anything else that evades us or that seems to be absent from our lives. It may be our justification for the areas in which we fail in life. Or, it may be the reason we lean on for not trying to complete a particular goal. The truth, however, may be that we are terrified to change our lives. We are afraid to try and live a truly joyous life. Develop your own positive and negative chart and analyze what you list. Can you identify your thought patterns? What can you do to start dispelling your long-held convictions?[36]

---

[36] Ibid.

Make a deliberate decision to adapt and to be fully responsible for your choices. Life is all about the power to choose. **Choose** to think positively. Make a resolution to amend old assumptions that may no longer apply. Be proactive and participate in your life rather than be a spectator. Taking that stand means managing your life in all ways. You are in charge of the food you eat, when you eat, and the judgements you have about the events that take place in your world. It is okay to consume something that you have been trying to avoid. Just remind yourself that you made up your mind to eat it. Don't beat yourself up over it. More importantly, don't allow it to derail your progress or stop you altogether. I heard a saying long ago that I never forgot, "It is okay to go off the road, just don't build a house." Acknowledge your decisions and get back on track.

THE BLAME GAME

I don't know about you, but when things get difficult, my first response is to find a reason that it's not my fault. It's hard feeling responsible all the time, and sometimes I feel that if I take myself out of the equation, then it's the people, the environment, or the circumstances taking place around me that *make* change impossible. Others cannot make us do something we are not willing to do. There will always be temptations. The trap is believing that outside forces are the problem. That you are a victim of your external environment.

I recall being in my early twenties and struggling to be happy. I was growing increasingly anxious about life in general and trying to place blame on my father for my predicament. During one conversation I pointed my finger at him accusing him of being the cause of my anxiety problem. He was not about to accept blame. He let me know it. He responded to my accusation by expressing, "Maybe I didn't do everything right, but I did the best I could. You are an adult now. You figure it out." I remember being so angry with him. How could he say that to me? After all, he is one of the primary people who raised me. Of course, I wanted him to be at fault for "messing me up." It took me a long time to get over the sting of those words and instead come to appreciate them. My reality is my responsibility. My life and how I handle my experiences belong to me. I could continue blaming someone outside, or I could take ownership and reclaim my life.

What's more important is that this interaction with my dad taught me to use my experiences for self-improvement. This exchange provoked some awareness, maybe for the first time, about *my* behaviors. Projecting outward was my response to my inner pain. I didn't want to feel it, so I tried to force it on someone else — in this case my father. It was an unconscious knee-jerk reaction. He just happened to be the one who was conveniently in the line of fire. I was not ready to take responsibility for my own well-being — my emotional well-being. I was attempting to dodge my responsibility for my emotional life at that time. I was either incapable of or possibly just unwilling to, admit what I was doing to avoid taking ownership.

We frequently search outside of ourselves expecting others or objects to fill whatever void we need filled. I heard what my father said to me. It made perfect sense after I had time to reflect. At the time, however, it felt like cold water was thrown on me because I was being challenged. I wasn't prepared for that. It was one of many wake-up calls. I didn't exactly know how to handle it. How would I solve my problem? How would I learn to find my own contentment? How would I muster up the courage to change?

While it took quite a bit of time for his statement to sink in and be truly understood, the seed was planted. That exchange would become one of the foundational experiences on which I would draw to make permanent changes in my thought process. You have your own distinctive life experiences that you can use as a springboard to transform your life. Basically, your life experiences are your mentors and are there to assist in your metamorphosis. Become cognizant of your inner world and watch how you evolve.

Looking back, I realize now that was actually the most loving thing my father could have done. He prompted me to think about the direction I wanted for my life. I had to come face-to-face with the fact that I control my life's destiny. You will need to come to terms with the fact that you control yours. I was in a tug-of-war between the desire to remain a child with others being responsible for my life and being an adult who is responsible for herself. It was no doubt easier to make my dad the scapegoat for the difficulty I was encountering. What good would that have done for me? He can't live my life for me, and the only reason I could think of wanting him to do that is that he would be the cause of failure, not me if life didn't turn out how I wanted. Looking back, I was petrified of taking control of my life. There is that fear again! Resolving inner conflict doesn't occur quickly, but it is necessary in all facets of life.

THE TALE OF TWO WOLVES

There is a Cherokee parable that depicts the emotional struggle associated with all aspects of human existence that I turn to again and again when I am feeling conflicted or at odds. It reads as follows:

> *An old Cherokee is teaching his grandson about life. "A fight is going on inside me," he said to the boy. "It is a terrible fight and it is between two wolves. One is evil—he is anger, envy, sorrow, regret, greed, arrogance, self-pity, guilt, resentment, inferiority, false pride, superiority and ego."*
>
> *He continued, "The other is good—he is joy, peace, love, hope, serenity, humility, kindness,*

benevolence, empathy, generosity, truth, compassion, and faith. The same fight is going on inside you—and inside every other person, too."

The grandson thought about it for a minute and then asked his grandfather, "Which wolf wins?"

The old Cherokee simply replied, "The one you feed."[37]

Acknowledging the existence of an ongoing internal battle of emotions that exists in all of us will be helpful in combating the critical sides of ourselves that berate our efforts and tell us we are undeserving of what we want to attain in life. I come to view the conflict within me as an interchange of ideas and information between my ego and my higher self. According to *the Holistic Psychologist*: "The ego is the "I." It is how you see yourself. It is the part of your mind that identifies with traits, beliefs, and habits. Your ego is an unconscious part of your mind."[38] The ego is the part of us that invented the story about ourselves, wants us to stay small and in familiar surroundings, too scared to make changes or

---

[37]"The Cherokee Two Wolves Story and the Power of Mindset," Clarity Clinic, Oct. 16, 2020, https://www.claritychi.com/the-cherokee-two-wolves-story-and-the-power-of-mindset/.

[38] N. "How to Do Ego Work." *The Holistic Psychologist*, May 17, 2019, https://theholisticpsychologist.com/how-to-do-ego-work/.

take chances. The higher self is our conscious self or our self of awareness. It is the part of ourselves that recognizes awareness. It is the self of all possibilities if we are willing to venture into the unknown. A great deal of our growth will come from identifying and deconstructing the stories that we created about ourselves. Get in touch with your inner script, and ask yourself if you are happy with the side of you that is winning the war. If the answer is no, then it's time to take the road less travelled and see where it leads.

Separating myself into two different identities: one as the thinker (the ego) and the other as the observer (the higher self) is a way that I have come to differentiate between my thoughts. The observer is the one who *witnesses* your thoughts and actions. It points out your nonsense and attempts to guide you down the right path by notifying you about how it feels about what you are doing. The problem is we don't have faith in that inner voice. Consequently, we often ignore it. We allow our egoic minds to override this intuition. Think of the observer as a "parental" figure that is always with you attempting to escort you lovingly along life's path with only the best intentions. The ego identity is the part of you carrying on like an unruly child. In a manner of speaking, the "parent" part of your consciousness needs to teach the "child" in you a more productive way to behave.

Let's look at a simple example. You've decided that you want to lose weight. You are getting off to a good start following a meal plan. You find yourself in a situation at work where you are working long hours to help out while a coworker is out on medical leave. Keeping up the pace is challenging. Your resistance is down because you are tired of working long hours. You decide to "treat" yourself to your favorite food because "you deserve it"—this is the ego talking. The ego will justify immediate gratification every time, even if the decision is not in the interest of supporting your weight loss goals. The observer part of you will recognize what the ego mind is telling you. This inner voice will remind you of how far you have come and how well your diet is going. It will suggest that you keep on your path rather than deviating for the momentary pleasure of a particular food. It is your inner guidance system providing counsel. I know you have experienced what I have illustrated. It's difficult to follow reason when your self-restraint is weakened. It is easier to make the choice that will make you feel better in the moment. I am not suggesting that it is wrong to eat the food if that is what you choose to do, but I am encouraging you to be open to what your inner self is trying to convey. After all, you will not get what you want if you always give in to your ego. Following your observer's sound advice is not easy. If you are consistent over time, however, it will become your best friend. It is your choice, and everything I've been trying to teach you in this book is about how having the information you need to make good choices makes you powerful.

CHAPTER NINE: SOME LAST THOUGHTS ON YOUR JOURNEY AND MINE

You, Janet, and I have been on a long journey over the course of this book. We've delved into the ways that your childhood shaped you, the ways that you have tried and failed to accomplish your goals in the past, and the ways that the Meal Wheel will put the power to succeed in your hands. We've hacked the way your body works to help you figure out what you can eat, and how to enjoy eating(!) to fuel your body while you lose excess weight. We've explored some ways that your spiritual and emotional life can support your goals in weight loss, and beyond weight loss. I've shared a lot about my life, and how my own spiritual life has helped me reach many of my goals.

A CONDUIT WITH A MESSAGE

I am a self-proclaimed seeker of the meaning of my life and I search for answers and direction in almost everything I encounter. Music has done a great deal to shape my world. British philosopher Alan Watts, once said that "music is one of the most spiritual of the arts because of its transient nature." It is played and then goes off into the ether remaining intangible as it disappears. We cannot touch or see the music, but there are parts that reverberate deep within us and remain there long after the music has stopped.

I have a propensity, at times, to take words too literally which has caused me unnecessary agony. Listening to songs, however, has always been a way to lift my spirits. These communications are pertinent to my emotional and spiritual development. How many times have you listened to a song and the meaning of it leaves an impression on you? How many times have you listened to a song and the message completely escaped you, but then you hear it again and you're left in awesome wonder? The song "Freewill" by Rush is one of those songs for me. It deals with our freedom to choose. These lyrics have helped me understand parts of my life that have been hard for me to accept.

This song literally brings tears to my eyes telling me that I would benefit from listening to what says. It screams, "Robin, open up your mind. Your life is now. Let go of what you need to let go of and get on with things!" Life is not a bunch of aimless experiences which we have no control over. Whether we realize it or not, we participate in every aspect of the life we live. Everything has meaning for one's own development. We must become aware of what we need to work on in order to succeed. Then, everything else will start to come together.

As I write this book, I am starting to think that while we experience different life situations, these experiences all lead to similar learning points. The song "Freewill" illustrates just about everything that I have felt or done. It offers a way out of the maze.

We can blame. We can give in to the fears that exist in our minds. We can avoid making the decision to change. We can chase after all the illusory happiness the world offers us through materialism. We can believe that the hand that we were dealt is the end of our road. Or, we can choose personal autonomy. How are these musicians able to compose such profound musical lyrics? Do they know something we don't know? Is the Universe using them as a conduit to help other individuals understand how to go beyond their irrational egoic selves that trap them? Personally, I have been guilty of succumbing to each of the thoughts described in that song. The song tells us that you can either keep yourself down or pull yourself up merely by making the choice to *think* differently. Everything is constructed first in our minds. Remove the shackles of your mind. Choose clarity and self-determination to create the life you want!

Encouragement can come from anywhere. Look for the positive meaning in everything! I think I have learned to do this out of sheer necessity otherwise I would have a hard time living. It is incredibly difficult to stay positive all of the time. I do not expect that you will. You can pay attention, however, to the contrasting moments when you ebb and flow in and out of a more positive state. When the gravity of negativity is pulling you down have ways to bring them up.

Let me share a story about how important I believe it is to have an optimistic mindset. There is a park near my home where

I frequently walk my dog. On several occasions, I found rocks that were painted with words of inspiration. I assume the rocks were strategically placed throughout the park with the intention that someone would find them. Each of the rocks that I found was inscribed with a different quote like, "You Rock", "Be You", "Lucky You", "Wipe the Slate Clean" and "Love". Most people would probably walk right past these rocks. I picked up every one of them on my travels as I felt they were meant for me. I believe that I found them to encourage me on my journey. I feel incredibly lucky to have found them as foolish as that may sound. My plan is to return them to the park when I no longer feel that I need their inspiration. Hopefully, they will uplift and motivate the next individual who finds them. Look around. Everything you need is right there. The Universe wants to see you flourish. You just need to have faith!

Making healthy food choices can also be life-affirming. Good food not only nourishes the body, it also improves your mood. Food has energy. Consuming nutritious food provides us with more potential to feel good both physically and emotionally. I love to start my day with a green shake consisting of baby spinach, pineapple, mango, banana, strawberries, and water. Everything is measured out to keep me within my carbohydrate designation. The hydrating shake is filled with antioxidants and provides a great start to my day. Nutritious high-energy foods are in their natural, whole state and include all fruits, vegetables, whole grains, herbal teas, nuts, seeds, monounsaturated oils, and legumes. Low-nutrition, low-energy foods include processed, packaged, and canned foods, white rice and flour, sugar, soda, coffee, alcohol, meat, fish and poultry, saturated fats, pasteurized dairy, and fried foods. Picking and choosing your foods wisely has the power to sustain your mind, body, and soul.[39]

Outside with my dog, spending time alone, painting, and visiting my family all raise my energy level as well. I do these activities as often as possible to maintain a positive outlook. Discover what uplifts your spirits and make time, but be careful what you choose. Purchasing another item of clothing, eating a favorite dessert, or participating in any type of addictive behavior are means used to take attention away from ourselves. They produce an illusion of momentary happiness, but they cannot provide any significant lasting meaning in our lives. We partake in these pastimes because we are trying to feel better. These behaviors represent our attempts to use external means to cope with internal distress or discontent. The feelings of pleasure will be fleeting. You will slip back down to a lower energy level as the initial effects subside. Essentially, you will need to buy more or eat more to feel better the next time. It is a vicious cycle. You can,

---

[39] Maria Benardis. "Eating High-Vibrational Foods for Good Health and Longevity." *Huffington Post*, Jun. 17, 2015, https://www.huffpost.com/entry/eating-high-vibrational-f_b_7596472.

however, get out of the loop. Build a strong inner foundation and the need for instant gratification will dissipate.

By turning your attention inward to find a more permanent solution to happiness you will find it easier to stay focused on your primary goals. You will eliminate distractions in the process. Seeking out ways to balance your inner self will also produce better long-term results which will affect your life beyond your weight loss goals. Achieving this requires spending time alone to get to know yourself. Feeling better will not only help you mentally and physically, but it will also make your surroundings more joyful.

CONTINUED HABITS

The blame game continued for me longer than I care to admit. Well beyond the incident with my father. It wasn't until I was in my mid-thirties that I was able to establish enough clarity around my thoughts that I could put a stop to blaming others. In 2006 I made the decision to go back to school and obtain a Master's in Business Administration. An MBA was a long-time goal, but I kept procrastinating. I finally applied and was accepted into Moravian University's MBA program. I was on my way to putting another check mark on my bucket list when I experienced, what I considered, some irrational anger issues.

I had a grueling schedule. I went to work for eight hours a day and then two nights a week I went to class from six to nine.

Sometimes I did not get an opportunity to eat dinner. All too frequently I was coming home hungry and tired. I started taking it out on my boyfriend. My anger got so bad that I found myself getting intensely irritated and frustrated on the drive home. I would deliberately start a fight with him as soon as I walked in the door. My attacks had nothing to do with him. The last time I launched into an argument with him I was once again pointing my finger and saying my usual, "you, you, you" and condemning him for basically being at home relaxing with the dog. Then I heard my inner voice shouting, "It's you, Robin. It's you. It's you." I was startled, but I realized I was projecting, once again, my frustrations onto an innocent bystander. My boyfriend has always been very kind in the way he communicates with me. He would say, "Listen, Robin, if you want to get a graduate degree that's great, and I will support you every step of the way. But if you don't want to do it then just stop. You can't keep coming home and taking it out on me. You have to make up your mind." Our internal battles can be so insidious that they can permeate into every aspect of life. I was working very hard to achieve my goal. Yet, I felt jealous of what I perceived as my boyfriend's freedom (or my perceived lack of freedom). I experienced these feelings even though it was my choice to go back to school. Again, it is the internal conflict where we form two different goals at the same time: being home with my family and going to graduate school. Of course, it is always more convenient to follow the easier path, but that path may not support your development. If you play the victim, you risk staying the victim.

I reflected on the position I had put my father in years ago. The incident with my dad was an early glimpse at my mental and emotional awakening. I thought I was over it. I thought I had it figured out. I have learned over the years that trapped negative emotions don't always disappear at this first recognition. We may "wake up" over and over again only to "fall asleep" in between incidents. This is part of the process. You get better at self-awareness the more you recognize your behaviors. This is part of maturing. Eventually, your negative thought patterns will dissolve one by one.

I have had similar experiences with patients who have said to me, "What are you going to do to get me to lose weight?" In other words, how are **you** going to correct **my** problem? The patients are not necessarily blaming me, but they want me to take on their dilemma. We may project the emotions that we don't want to or can't bear to accept in ourselves onto those around us. That was what I was doing to my father and my boyfriend. Our hurdles in life are sometimes like hot stones. We want to get rid of them quickly and we don't really care who we throw them at as long we distance them from ourselves. There are some problems in life that, as much as we may want to rid ourselves of them, belong to us (at least temporarily). If we can systematically start transforming them, we are on the path to possibly removing them completely. If we ignore them, we risk greater suffering. Most patients are receptive to my gentle, but firm, approach of putting the hot stone back in their lap. I will point out what they said. Ultimately, they need to listen to their inner thoughts and the words they speak. Some need to understand that their words and ideas are self-defeating. Some people have laughed when I repeat back what they said to me because they hear the foolishness of their words. I can relate to them because I have done it. We become so programmed to our own deluded thinking that we don't hear the insanity of our rhetoric. Your will to succeed must override the obstacles that reside inside you. Be willing to listen to the lack of reason streaming through your head. Be strong enough to shut it down so you can reach your goals.

WALKING THROUGH KARMA

The word Karma in Sanskrit means "act" or "action" and refers to a cycle of cause and effect—actions and the consequences of those actions. Karma is dynamic in nature and can be changed anytime through our own volition. Karma is influenced by both ***thoughts*** and ***actions***. What you do now will have some future impact. The way it is frequently used today has negative connotations attached to it because it is viewed as a punishment for some wrongdoing but, that is not how it works. According to Barbara O'Brien, journalist, and student of Zen Buddhism, karma is defined as follows:

> "In Buddhism, karma is an energy created by willful action through thoughts, words, and deeds. We are all creating karma every minute, and the

> karma we create affects us every minute. It's common to think of "my karma" as something you did in your last life that seals your fate in this life, but this is not Buddhist understanding. You can change the course of your life right now by changing your intentional acts and self-destructive patterns."[40]

My road to developing awareness around my thoughts has differed from many of the stories I've read. I did not have a single traumatic experience awaken me. Rather, I have experienced a string of events at various junctures in my life. Through allowing myself to explore my responses to these life events, I have been able to grow. My learning curve has been slow and steady and, often, troublesome. Patience has been a good friend. It will be a good friend to you on your journey. There have been moments when I really felt I had a good grasp on my emotions only to backslide into what I call negative sleepwalking time and time again. A good example of this is the blame habit. I recognized what I was doing, but I continued to do it until one day I accepted my thought process and my actions. Then it really sunk in. It was going to keep happening until I learned what my role was in the

---

[40] Lachlan Brown, "Karma definition: Most people are wrong about the meaning," Ideapod, May 1, 2021. https://ideapod.com/heres-great-explanation-karma-really-means-can-improve-life/

situation. Life is a big learning curve. I've never been able to get too settled before another challenge arises.

Roadblocks are all too common. Just as I surpass one barrier another barrier seems to be waiting for me. I have become quite adept at identifying obstructions in my life. While it may take me some time to overcome these impediments, I continue to work through them every day. My method of looking at the hindrances in my life has enabled me to master them. For instance, I no longer take offense as easily as I used to. It's not personal. The problem is present for my greater good whether I like it or not. I now feel more comfortable with the concept that the limit is actually something that my mind has set. Second, I try to allow myself to listen to my feelings about the event even though I may not like what I sense. Third, I act so that I begin to feel better. Repetition is necessary for permanent change. My methods have developed over the years. I encourage you to take measures to heal yourself from the inside.

It's only recently that I started piecing the different aspects of my life together to have a better understanding of what it all means for me, the life I am living, and the life to which I aspire. Looking back on the barriers I have overcome as well as the challenges that I face in the present, I have developed confidence that there is a purpose to everything that happens. If you examine your life events, you will be able to make more sense of your path and what learning points are meant for you. You may understand your struggles in a new way. By changing your perspective, you may find it easier to prevail.

Remember that I told you about beginning to work with an energy healer/coach? It's been a life-changing experience. I am looking at my world through a new set of eyes. She has helped me to appreciate the events in my life in ways I would never have been able to do on my own. Her response to an event I shared with her was, "Do you know what that was? You walked through karma." That statement validated my feelings as it meant that I had overcome an excruciating difficulty. In a manner of speaking, I paid a karmic debt-- changing a repetitive behavior or way of thinking so that it no longer had a negative influence on my life. Having a better understanding of what karma means and the ability to apply it to my life in a meaningful way has altered my path. My life puzzle is starting to come together. I will attempt to share my observations of this moment hoping that it will provide insight into your life.

I had, what I consider to be, a happy childhood. I was loved. My physical needs were met. As an adult, however, I questioned if my emotional needs as a child were given adequate attention. Being more sensitive than my older sibling, I required more encouragement and reinforcement. I am sure that my parents did their best, but most likely they did not receive the benefits of psychological support. Consequently, they were unable to provide me with what I needed. I have had a hard time accepting this lack of emotional support. I no longer look at my past, however, as a burden, but rather an opportunity. Currently, I accept that life is a continuous pursuit of resolutions. Maybe someone did not provide you with something that you needed. Now what? There is no going back. Others can no longer make up for what they did not know how to provide initially. Recall my blame game? You have two options. Remain unhappy in the negative place you are in or choose to look at your behavior and then take corrective action. I have replaced frustration with determination. I am solving my problems.

My life prior to college graduation outwardly appeared happy and uneventful. I was painfully shy, but I partook in the usual childhood activities -- going to school, participating in sports, and maintaining friendships. Somewhere along my path, I developed a belief that everything I did had to be perfect. I wouldn't miss a day of school. I strove for straight A's. I also became very rigid in my thinking. This inflexibility worked fine when everything was going well. But we must remember that life doesn't always go smoothly. Some events made me feel worse than others, but I always persevered. I was a strong athlete, but I began to dislike the competition because I didn't have complete control over the outcome or how it made me feel if I didn't perform well. My self-esteem was not great, and perfectionism only made things more difficult.

Looking back on my childhood I have come to understand

how some of my negative feelings began. Others have completely eluded me. During my college senior year, I developed an anxiety disorder. I was confused as to why I found myself in that situation so late in my schooling. As my college years ended, my emotional state began to unravel. I became so anxious I could barely sit through a class. My mind would ruminate on my anxious feelings only to compound them. I began missing classes which eventually affected my final grades. I developed crippling anxiety which seemingly came out of nowhere. I was able to finish my last semester and graduate. Then my real education began.

The anxiety was very pervasive. I eventually had a hard time being around people. Going to the local pharmacy to buy gum caused severe angst. I describe the feeling as wanting to crawl out of my skin and run away. Run away to where? I didn't know. What I did know was that I didn't want to feel the pain of my anxiety. I thought that I could manage it on my own. I was under the impression that avoidance was a feasible option but I was mistaken. I didn't realize that the only way out of this crisis was to face it, to feel it. And to do that, I would need to enlist help.

This situation escalated and I went to my mother to ask for help. The assistance that I wanted was in the form of medication to numb my suffering. My mother listened to me and scheduled an appointment with a psychologist. She even brought me to the visit. The psychologist asked me to explain what was troubling me, and I told her. After a brief discussion, she said, "I think you would benefit from group therapy." I, of course, disagreed. I asked her if she could prescribe an anti-anxiety medication. She told me she did not have prescription privileges. I became annoyed by her response. I was upset that I could not get the immediate relief that I was seeking. I got up and stormed out of the office. Once back at the car, I told my mother, "I will get over this on my own." While a door had slammed in my face and I felt alone, I developed a sense of determination. I decided to work on it alone. But I had no idea what to do or how difficult the journey would be. The anger I felt from being denied my request ignited something in me. I was not certain how to proceed and there was no plan to manage this problem. Memories from my childhood, however, resonated that it was not an option to feel sorry for myself. I took the only action I knew and I pressed on which turned out to be a very lengthy and painful process. Looking back, however, I wouldn't have it any other way.

Putting myself in the most uncomfortable situations proved to be the key to overcoming my anxiety. I even went back to school. This was extremely challenging because I had no choice but to sit in a classroom full of people for an hour and a half. It was agonizing. Finding ways to cope with unpleasant feelings became my mission. Sitting by doors, windows, and heaters proved helpful. The noise from the heaters distracted my mind from going wild. My focus was always on how to distance myself from my thoughts. I was functioning strictly in a survival mode.

Sadly, I thought I might have to live like this forever, but I kept confronting my fear. I honestly didn't know what else I could do. I still had to live my life. At that time, I was also working with a therapist to help me work through my distress. Then, one day, my anxiety disappeared. It vanished as quickly as it arrived.

The consequences of perfectionism, self-criticism, and the need to control had caught up to me and manifested as severe anxiety. I did not intentionally set out to heal this part of myself, but that is what ended up happening. I understand, now, that I connected my self-worth to the opinions and acceptance of my family. I reacted to statements such as, "B+…why wasn't it an A?" or "Blend in" by feeling inadequate. Comments like that can be demoralizing especially when you are young and impressionable. They end up shaping our beliefs about ourselves and those beliefs keep us from moving forward.

I recognize that my way may not work for everyone. Everyone's experience with anxiety is different. Through my unique journey, I was able to improve my self-efficacy and gain confidence in my ability to participate in the world. I learned that I was good enough. Thinking back, you would have been hard-pressed to get me to admit that I had poor self-esteem. That would be difficult for almost anyone to admit. Had I been able to face that reality sooner I would have suffered less.

During this time, I came to accept that nothing terrible was going to happen. I was learning how to control my mind. I was in the process of dispelling the defeatist beliefs that I allowed to reside in my mind for too long. I realized my anxiety was trying to communicate to me that my belief system was out of alignment — wrong thinking. My mental insecurities were manifesting outwardly as anxiety and fear. I could not see past that fear. I was able to endure for the time necessary for my subconscious to accept and change. The old thoughts were no longer a threat. I am happy to say that I have not experienced anything even remotely like that anxiety again.

Debilitating anxiety was not my karma. It was, however, an outward manifestation of a maladaptive thought process. My karma was permitting the same negative thoughts repeatedly to run my life. It was habitual. I could not escape myself. I can now say with great certainty that my inner mindset of varying degrees of unworthiness, doubt, shame, and fear created my anxiety. I had to feel the uneasiness of those emotions to get over them. This is how karma gets passed down. Generations just keep the same beliefs alive. That's why it's up to each individual to break the karma through new thoughts and actions.

Standing in physical discomfort day after day for years is not what I would suggest anyone do as most people would not tolerate suffering for very long. It is clear why people get addicted to a myriad of activities and substances to repress their feelings. I wanted medication. I also experienced times when I thought alcohol could be the best method of calming myself. Then, I heard my inner voice tell me, "You don't want to go down that rabbit hole, Robin." Thankfully, I chose to listen to those wise words.

These are my memories generated out of sheer desperation. I can relate to how easily it is to lose control of your mind and then have it control you. It happens unexpectedly. Before you know it, you have a much bigger problem. There are many other ways to cope while learning how to succeed in dealing with inner barriers. I followed my own route and came to my own conclusions. I also began to have more faith in listening to my intuition to shepherd my decision-making. I can tell you that it works. I now see the bigger picture. I can say confidently, "Yes, I walked through karma."

Having gone through a release of some of my negative karma, I now embrace my personal problems, or my "subconscious bucket list", with the sole purpose of expanding my true nature. As previously mentioned, my anxiety was not my karma, and your distress is not yours. Anxiety and distress are examples of outward signals that we must realign to correct thinking. We need to turn our focus inward. The same old behaviors and the way we repeatedly speak to ourselves, reinforcing wrong thinking, are the karma from which we must break free. We tend to put emphasis on the wrong issues. It's no wonder that change is a difficult task. My switch in perspective has allowed me to work on absolving the negative energy that holds me back rather than resenting it and causing me to remain at a standstill.

I feel as if I am in the process of walking through karma again. The recent pandemic has redirected my priorities. I am happy to have had the opportunity to slow down and reflect. If that didn't take place, I would still be doing the exact same thing I was doing previously with very little impetus to better myself or even push myself into my life's purpose.

I never worried about losing my job before COVID. In fact, everyone always told me that I would have my job for as long as I wanted. When COVID-19 emerged, I became extremely fearful of losing my financial lifeline. I convinced myself that my job was going to be dismantled and parts would be given away to other people. I envisioned a real crisis that would set me on a whole new life path, but not on my terms.

During this period, I actually felt the fire to get this book completed. Nothing like the threat of a loss of income to move you to act. I found it disappointing, though, that the fear of losing something caused me to act. I shared my worries with a friend who told me, "You won't lose your job. Why would you think about doing something else? You have a great job that pays well and has good benefits." When I heard her words my first thought was yes, it is a good job and it has served me well. My next thought, however, was that I had outgrown it. More importantly, why did I think it's the best I can do? What if there was something more that I could do to share my knowledge, both professional and personal, with others to help them on their journey? What was stopping me from completing this project? It was the same familiar state of mind that held me back from just about everything — fear that maybe the book would not be any good or that people would hate it. I translated that to mean, "I'm not good enough" or "What if people don't like me." Same old negative thoughts. Yes, I can choose to take up permanent residence here. But I am not sure I want to. Does this sound familiar? Ask yourself what is fueling your recurring attitudes toward your situation. What is stopping you from achieving your goals? Do you have a sense that you could do more? What does your intuition tell you? Are there measures that you would take if you weren't getting in your own way?

My thoughts have a definitive pattern. I suspect you will discover your patterns once you start creating awareness around the negative constructs of your mind. Mine circled back to conquering my thoughts around my own values. The mind is like a garden. If you don't tend to it regularly, the weeds of negativity take over. Practice planting positive seeds and then hone in on controlling the negative ones that have grown a home. It's hard to tell from where all of our negative seeds arise. Maybe they came from words that people said to us, or actions they took toward us over the years, or perhaps from ways we witnessed people behave with each other. Perhaps they were things that were meant to caution a whole class at school, or us and all of our siblings and we took them too personally. As children, we don't know any better than to be hurt by someone's callousness. I took a lot to heart when I was younger because I didn't know how to separate my emotional baggage from someone else's. I find comfort in that I am getting better at identifying my negative repressed emotions. The scars on my psyche will always remain. Breaking away from our negative thought patterns is difficult. One option is to revise your original script. It's one way of breaking your cycle, but I am sure it is not the only way. I think we can all agree, however, that it's time to move on.

TOUGH LOVE

Hindsight really is 20/20! It turns out that my family provided me with the physical and emotional environment essential for my emotional and spiritual growth, even if the presentation was unpleasantly rough at times. It was their job to keep me safe, provide advice to help me problem solve, and raise me to be a competent individual who can function independently. The baton was passed. It is now my job to take these skills and resolve my issues on my own. Not everyone is brought up being taught how to solve their own problems. It may be beneficial to dedicate some time to educating yourself on healthy discernment and problem-solving. I have spent a significant amount of time researching ways to settle inner conflict which my family did not teach me. In fact, I have come to the conclusion that while we have many relationships to help us on our path, life is primarily an individual journey. There is much that you will need to discover on your own. This journey of discovery is truly wonderful.

The stage has been set for you. Your life has provided you with the specific circumstances vital to your development. All you have to do is adjust your outlook about how you were raised, who did you wrong, how you failed in the past, your unfortunate lot in life, your crummy job, your unsatisfying relationship, etc. You get the picture. I have spent years harboring resentments and complaining about those individuals closest to me. Yet, here I am disclosing my revelations to you.

We are primarily responsible for how our life unfolds. Even when circumstances beyond your control occur, you direct how you think about them and how you approach them. We may exhibit negative resistance along the way. I find, however, that it is the resistance that makes our problems persist. I am doing much better since I adopted and employed new strategies for taking charge of my life. A little trick that has helped me is that I ask myself, in any situation, What is my role? What am I feeling? Why do I feel this way? Why am I reacting this way? Why am I avoiding change? What can I do to make this situation better? Rather than looking outside of myself, I find myself saying, "Oh, it's me again." I bring it back to me. At first, this was difficult because I didn't like seeing the uglier negative side of myself. The side that is argumentative, angry, blames, complains, points out other's shortcomings, wants everything to be easy. I am now more relaxed with this exercise. I realize that I can change myself. I can't change what is outside of me — including other people.

There is an infomercial that I am only able to tolerate listening to the first couple of sentences before I shut it off. The gentleman says, "It's not your fault if you can't make good food choices because the restaurants are making unhealthy food and marketing it to you." He very well may go on to say something very profound, but he loses me immediately. This broadcast is a classic example of what people are up against. Only if you allow it, will marketing complicate matters when it comes to adhering to a meal plan. The minute your ego sees any opportunity to defend its position it starts saying, "You are right. It is not my fault." Your job, however, is to recognize and understand what your mind is doing and put to stop to it immediately.

Nobody can make healthy choices for you. The food industry is in the business of producing food that people enjoy and will purchase. They market to our desires knowing that we usually buy what we want. Marketers understand that people have a difficult time controlling their minds. Marketers are free to do what they want (within legal parameters) just as you are. The food industry is not responsible for our health just as other businesses are not responsible for our happiness. In the past, I have fallen victim to believing material things will make me happy. If you accept the idea that something or someone outside is responsible for your decisions then you will suffer disappointment. I have had to work very hard to shift my frame of reference. I am only trying to help shift your perceptions to expand your awareness.

We live in a diverse environment where we are bombarded with endless amounts of external stimuli that we must process in order to make the best decisions. This is not an easy task. Time and time again various factors try to influence our choices. Ask yourself: What am I feeling right now? Why do I want this food? Why is it hard for me to make a healthier food choice? Don't give your power away to the marketers. Your power to choose is the greatest resource that you have. If you master the art of choosing wisely, you will be able to move confidently through life and adhere to your diet.

SOME LAST QUESTIONS FOR YOU:

- Have you recognized that setting and meeting this goal is difficult, but that you are up to the challenge? What are your fears? How do the tools we've discussed here help you to overcome those fears?
- What does it feel like to know that you've demonstrated a lot of commitment by deciding that this is the right time for you to lose weight? What does that say to you about who you are?
- What is your support network? (this book, friends, family members) How will you ask them to support you? How will you ask them to help you when you plateau or backslide? How will you ask for support when you feel

like giving up?

- What is your plan for when you "fail" (by skipping workouts, "cheating," backsliding)? How will you forgive yourself and start again?
- How will you reward yourself for your success in ways that support your new lifestyle?
- What does your life look like when you achieve your goal? How has working (and succeeding) on your weight loss goals inspired you to take action in other areas of your life?

FINAL THOUGHTS

American author Neale Donald Walsch said:

> "I discovered that ninety-eight percent of the world's people spend ninety-eight percent of their time on things that don't matter. That is, most people are unaware of their true purpose and identity. They mistakenly believe life is just a series of milestones: finding love, getting a job, getting the kids, getting the corner office, getting a bigger house and eventually growing old and getting the hell out. That's not what life is about. People are stuck on autopilot, blindly following a script that's been written for them."[41]

---

[41] *E-Motion*, directed by Frazer Bailey (2014: Play Pictures), DVD.

So often, we seemingly get everything we want, but still are not satisfied. We go through life looking at it at face value rather than digging for the deeper meaning. We are often left feeling empty as if something is missing. We attempt to bypass doing the introspective work necessary to transform our lives. Avoidance, however, is rarely a feasible option. While people strive to accomplish everything that Neale Donald Walsch expresses, it's the emotions that we experience in response to those situations that are the key to our emancipation. Our stuck emotions are the barriers that need to be reconciled for us to experience the lives we want.

We all want to live a more joyous and fulfilling life. How we go about obtaining that life can be baffling. You are learning to communicate with your inner self. This communication will provide guidance on what is necessary for you to master. Begin to tap into your critical thinking side to determine the best approach to undo your knots. Everything you require to overcome any barrier is inside of you. You just have to call upon it. Remember, tackle the inner issues and the outside will take care of itself. Ultimately, if you can accomplish these activities, you will easily get what you want including weight loss!

Picking up this book may prove to be the first step toward recognizing the thoughts and beliefs that are keeping you from progressing with your weight loss and perhaps even other areas of your life. You may find yourself uncomfortable with this process. You are not alone. Do not get discouraged and give up. Feel your discomfort and listen to it. The discomforting troubling feelings may give you some insight into your barriers. You may feel better just acknowledging that you have some feelings that accompany this undertaking.

SOME FINAL WORDS FROM JANET

About four years after I first met Janet, I received a bouquet of flowers and a card at my office. The card was a birthday card, which was funny because it wasn't anywhere near my birthday. Handwritten inside the card were these words from Janet:

Dear Robin,

It's my birthday (55 sounded pretty old when I was young, but now it feels like the start of a fabulous time) and I wanted to thank you for everything you taught me. I've had ups and downs on the scale, but ever since I first met you, I've felt as if I have had the power to take care of my health. I've been at a happy weight for more than a year, and I really feel like I am alive and healthy to celebrate this birthday because I stopped ignoring what my body was telling me, and took my health into my own hands.

Gratefully,

Janet

The Meal Wheel will help you with dietary practicalities. Just like Janet, you will use the tools to accomplish your goals. You will have challenges, backslides, supportive friends, and people who sabotage you. You will want to quit some days, and some days you will feel on top of the world. Adopting a healthier way of eating resulting in long-term, successful weight management must be accompanied by reflection on how you approach your life. This reflection will pave the way toward making improvements in all areas of your life. Remember, you can't always control outside events, but you can absolutely control your perception of and response to them! I know that you can succeed because I have helped lots of people to succeed using the same tools I've shared with you here. You deserve empathy, encouragement, and recognition that what you're doing is momentous. You deserve to have what you want from your life.

Wishing you good health,

Robin Gayle

APPENDIX

Appendix A

1,300 Calories (without snacks)

Breakfast 3 carbohydrate choices:	1) ½ cup cooked plain oatmeal (page 202)
	2) ½ cup cooked plain oatmeal (page 202)
	3) ¾ cup blueberries (page 204)
1 fat choice:	1) 4 walnut halves (page 210)
Lunch 3 carbohydrate choices:	1) 1 slice of whole grain bread (page 201)
	2) 1 slice of whole grain bread (page 201)
	3) 4 oz. yogurt (check the label)
2 oz lean protein:	1) 1 1/2 oz. turkey (page 209)
	2) ½ oz. cheese (page 209)
1 fat:	1) 1 tsp. mayonnaise (page 210)
Freebies:	Side salad with balsamic vinegar (page 208)
Dinner 3 carbohydrate choices:	1) ½ cup mashed potatoes (page 204)
	2) ½ cup peas or corn (page 203)
	3) 1 cup cubed cantaloupe (page 204)
3 oz lean protein:	1) 3 oz. baked chicken breast w/o skin (page 209)
1 fat:	1) 1 tsp. of butter to make the potato (page 211)
Freebies:	Side salad with balsamic vinegar (page 208)

1,300 Calories (with between-meal snacks)

Breakfast 2 carbohydrate choices:	1) 1 slice of whole grain bread (page 201)
	2) 1 ¼ cups whole strawberries (page 205)
1 fat:	1) 2 tsp. peanut butter (page 210)
Snack 1 carbohydrate choice:	1) 4 oz. yogurt (check the label)
Lunch 2 carbohydrate choices:	1) 2 slices of low-calorie bread (page 201)
	2) 1 small piece of fruit (page 204-206)
2 oz. lean protein:	1) 2 oz. tuna in water (page 209)
1 fat:	1) 1 Tbsp. low-fat mayonnaise (page 210)
Freebies:	Raw veggies with 1 Tbsp. fat-free dip (page 207-208)
Snack 1 carbohydrate choice:	1) ½ Nature Valley granola bar (check the label)
Dinner 2 carbohydrate choices:	1) 1/3 cup cooked brown rice (page 203)
	2) 1/3 cup cooked brown rice (page 203)
3 oz. lean protein:	1) 3 oz. seasoned pork tenderloin (page 209)
1 fat:	1) 1 tsp. butter (page 211)
Snack 1 carbohydrate choice:	1) 3 cups popcorn with spray butter (page 212)

1,400 Calories (without snacks)

Breakfast	
3 carbohydrate choices:	1) 1 1/2 cups unsweetened cereal (page 202)
	2) ½ cup 1% milk (page 207)
	3) ½ small banana (page 204)
1 fat:	1) 2 Tbsp. half & half (page 211)
Freebies:	Coffee or tea with artificial sweetener
Lunch	
3 carbohydrate choices:	1) 1 6-in. soft corn tortilla shell (page 202)
	2) ¼ cup refried beans (page 204)
	3) 1/3 cup cooked brown rice (page 203)
3 oz. lean protein:	1) 3 oz. grilled chicken breast (page 209)
2 fats:	1) 2 Tbsp. sour cream (page 211)
	2) ¼ avocado (page 210)
Freebies:	Tomato-based salsa, shredded lettuce, and tomatoes; salad with fat-free balsamic dressing (page 207-208)
Dinner	
3 carbohydrate choices:	1) 1/3 cup wheat pasta (page 203)
	2) 1/3 cup wheat pasta (page 203)
	3) 1/3 cup wheat pasta (page 203)
3 oz lean protein:	1) 3oz lean ground beef (page 209)
1 fat:	1) 1 Tbsp. regular salad dressing (page 211)
Freebies:	½ cup no-sugar-added tomato sauce; veggie salad (page 208)

1,400 Calories (with between-meal snacks)

Breakfast	
2 carbohydrate choices:	1) ½ English muffin (page 202)
	2) ¾ cup blackberries (page 204)
1 fat:	1) 2 tsp. peanut butter (page 210)
Snack	
1 carbohydrate choice:	1) 4 oz. yogurt (check the label)
Lunch	
2 carbohydrate choices:	1) ½ 6-in. pita (page 201)
	2) ½ 6-in. pita (page 201)
3 oz. lean protein:	1) 3 oz. cubed chicken breast (page 209)
2 fats:	1) 1 Tbsp. low-fat mayonnaise (page 210)
	2) 1 Tbsp. Ranch dressing (page 211)
Freebies:	Baby carrots; onion, and celery in chicken salad and a side salad (page 207-208)
Snack	
1 carbohydrate choice:	1) 1 small piece of fruit (page 204-205)
Dinner	
2 carbohydrate choices:	1) 1/3 cup cooked quinoa (page 203)
	2) 1/3 cup cooked quinoa (page 203)
3 oz. lean protein:	1) 3 oz. baked salmon (page 209)
1 fat:	1) 1 Tbsp. regular salad dressing (page 211)
Freebies:	1 cup asparagus and side salad with balsamic vinegar (page 207-208)
Snack	
1 carbohydrate choice:	1) ½ cup low-fat ice cream (check the label)

1,500 Calories (with evening snack)

Breakfast	
3 carbohydrate choices:	1) 1 slice of whole grain bread (page 201)
	2) 4 oz. yogurt (check the label)
	3) ¾ cup raspberries (page 205)
1 fat:	1) 1 Tbsp. avocado or guacamole (page 210)
Lunch	
3 carbohydrate choices:	1) 1/3 cup wheat angel hair pasta (page 203)
	2) 1/3 cup wheat angel hair pasta (page 203)
	3) 1/3 cup wheat angel hair pasta (page 203)
3 oz. lean protein:	1) 2 oz. grilled chicken breast (page 209)
	2) 1 oz. feta cheese (page 209)
2 fats:	1) 1 1/2 tsp. olive oil for pasta (page 210)
	2) 4 kalamata olives chopped in pasta (pg 210)
Freebies:	Artichoke hearts, grape tomatoes, lemon juice, and salt and pepper to mix with pasta (page 207-208)
Dinner	
3 carbohydrate choices:	1) ½ cup baked fries (page 203)
	2) ½ cup baked fries (page 203)
	3) 1/3 cup baked beans (page 203)
3 oz. lean protein:	1) 3 oz. lean burger (page 209)
2 fats:	1) 1 Tbsp. avocado (page 210)
	2) 1 Tbsp. avocado (page 210)
Freebies:	Lettuce, tomato, 1 Tbsp. ketchup (page 207-210)
Snack	
1 carbohydrate choice:	1) 2 small fat-free cookies (check the label)

1,500 Calories (with between-meal snacks)

Breakfast	
2 carbohydrates choices:	1) 1 whole grain waffle (page 202)
	2) 1 whole-grain waffle (page 202)
1 fat:	1) 2 tsp. peanut butter (page 210)
Freebie:	1 Tbsp. sugar-free jam
Snack	
1 carbohydrate choice:	1) 1 small piece of fruit (page 204-206)
Lunch	**Ham and Cheese Melt**
2 carbohydrate choices:	1) 1 cup tomato soup (check the label)
	2) 2 slices of low-calorie bread (page 201)
3 oz. lean protein:	1) 1 oz. ham (page 209)
	2) 2 oz. cheese (page 209)
2 fats:	1) 1 Tbsp. reduced-fat margarine (page 210)
	2) 2 Tbsp. low-fat salad dressing (page 211)
Freebies:	Vegetable side salad (page 207- 206)
Snack	
1 carbohydrate choice:	1) 1/3 cup hummus (page 203)
Freebie:	Red, yellow and green pepper, sliced (page 207)
Dinner	**Tacos**
2 carbohydrate choices:	1) 2 taco shells (page 201)
	2) ½ cup black beans (page 203)
3 oz. lean protein:	1) 2 oz. lean beef (page 209)
	2) 1 oz. shredded cheese (page 209)
2 fats:	1) ¼ avocado (page 210)
	2) 2 Tbsp. low-fat salad dressing (page 211)
Freebies:	Shredded lettuce and tomato for taco and a side salad (207-208)
Snack	
1 carbohydrate choice:	1) 1 fudge pop (check the label)

1,600 Calories (with evening snack)

Breakfast 3 carbohydrate choices:	1) ¾ cup bran flakes (page 202)
	2) 1 cup skim milk (page 207)
	3) 1 mediuml peach (page 205)
1 oz. lean protein:	1) ¼ cup low-fat cottage cheese (page 209)
Lunch	**Cheese Pizza**
3 carbohydrate choices:	1) 2 slices of thin-crust pizza (12-in. pie label)
2 oz. lean protein:	1) 2 oz shredded cheese on pizza (page 209)
2 fats:	1) 2 tsp. olive oil to make the pizza (page 210)
Freebies:	Side salad with balsamic vinegar; tomato sauce (page 207-208)
Dinner 4 carbohydrate choices:	1) 1 cup of cooked noodles (page 203)
	2) ½ cup applesauce (page 205)
3 oz protein:	1) 3 oz. lean pork (page 209)
2 fats:	1) 1 slice of bacon (page 211)
	2) 1 Tbsp. light margarine (page 210)
Freebie:	Cabbage (page 207)
Snack 1 carbohydrate choice:	1) 5 Saltine crackers (check label)
1 fat:	1) 1 Tbsp. cream cheese (page 211)
Freebie:	1 Tbsp. sugar-free jam

1,600 calories (with between-meal snacks)

Breakfast 2 carbohydrate choices: 1 oz. lean protein: 1 fat:	 1) 1 low-calorie English muffin (page 202) 2) ½ cup mixed fresh fruit (page 204-205) 1) 1 egg (page 209) 1) 1 Tbsp. low fat margarine (page 210)
Snack 1 carbohydrate choice:	 1) 4 oz. yogurt (label)
Lunch 3 carbohydrate choices: 2 oz. lean protein: 1 fat: Freebies:	 1) 1 wheat wrap (page 202) 2) ½ cup black beans and corn mix (page 203) 3) 10 tortilla chips (label) 1) 2 oz. ground turkey (page 209) 1) ¼ of an avocado (page 210) Diced tomatoes and shredded lettuce (page 208)
Snack 1 carbohydrate choice:	 1) 3 cups air-popped popcorn (page 212)
Dinner 3 carbohydrate choices: 3 oz. lean protein: 2 fats: Freebies:	**Stuffed Peppers** 1) 1/3 cup brown rice (page 203) 2) 1/3 cup brown rice (page 203) 3) 1/3 cup brown rice (page 203) 1) 3 oz. lean ground beef (page 209) 1) 1 tsp. olive oil (page 210) 2) 1 tsp. olive oil (page 210) Green bell pepper, onion, and tomato sauce for stuffing (page 205-208)
Snack 1 carbohydrate choice:	 1) 3 small figs or dates (page 206)

1,700 calories (without snacks)

Breakfast	
3 carbohydrate choices:	1) ½ cup cooked oatmeal (page 202)
	2) ½ cup cooked oatmeal (page 202)
	3) 1 small banana (page 203)
2 fats:	1) 4 walnut halves (page 210)
	2) 2 Tbsp. creamer (page 211)
Freebie:	1) Coffee with sugar substitute
Lunch	**Roast Beef and Cheese Sandwich**
4 carbohydrate choices:	1) 1 slice of wheat bread (page 201)
	2) 1 slice of wheat bread (page 201)
	3) 1 cup low-fat milk (page 207)
	4) ½ Nature Valley granola bar (label)
3 oz. lean protein:	1) 2 oz. lean roast beef (page 209)
	2) 1 oz. low-fat cheese (page 209)
2 fats:	1) 1 tsp. mayonnaise (page 210)
	2) 1 Tbsp. Ranch dressing (page 211)
Freebie:	1) 1 cup baby carrots (page 207)
Dinner	**Chili with Ground Turkey**
4 carbohydrates:	1) ½ cup turkey chili with beans (page 203)
	2) ½ cup turkey chili with beans (page 203)
	3) 1/3 cup brown rice (page 203)
	4) 1/3 cup brown rice (page 203)
5 oz. protein:	1) 4 oz. turkey in chili (page 209)
	2) 1 oz. low-fat shredded cheddar cheese (page 209)
1 fat:	1) 2 Tbsp. sour cream (page 211)
Freebie:	Side salad with balsamic vinegar (page 207-208)

1,700 calories (with between-meal snacks)

Breakfast	
3 carbohydrate choices:	1) ½ cup hash brown potatoes (page 204)
	2) 2 slices of wheat toast (page 203)
2 oz. lean protein:	1) 1 egg + 1 egg white (page 209)
	2) 1 oz. turkey sausage (for omelet) (page 209)
2 fats:	1) 2 tsp. butter (page 211)
	2) 1 Tbsp. creamer (page 211)
Freebies:	Coffee with artificial sweetener
Snack	
1 carbohydrate choice:	1) 1/3 cup hummus (page 203)
Freebie:	1) Grape tomatoes/baby carrots (pg 207-208)
Lunch	
3 carbohydrate choices:	1) 2 slices wheat bread (page 201)
	2) 1 small banana (page 204)
1 fat:	1) 2 tsp. nut butter (page 210)
Freebie:	Side salad with balsamic vinegar (page 207-208)
Snack	
1 carbohydrate choice:	1) 3 graham cracker squares (check the label)
	1) 3 cups plain popcorn with butter spray and pepper (page 212)
Dinner	
3 carbohydrate choices:	1) ½ cup mashed potatoes (page 204)
	2) ½ cup mashed potatoes (page 204)
	3) ½ cup applesauce (page 205)
6 oz. lean protein:	1) 6 oz. marinated pork tenderloin (page 209)
1 fat:	1) 1 Tbsp. blue cheese dressing (page 211)
Freebie:	Side salad with balsamic vinegar (page 208)

1,800 calories (without snacks)

Breakfast	
4 carbohydrate choices:	1) ½ cup cooked cream of wheat (page 202)
	2) ½ cup cooked cream of wheat (page 202)
	3) 1 medium peach (page 204)
	4). 4 oz. plain low-fat yogurt (page 207)
1 fat:	1) 2 Tbsp. creamer (page 211)
Freebie:	1) Coffee
Lunch	**Chicken Salad Sandwich**
4 carbohydrate choices:	1) 1 slice whole grain bread (page 201)
	2) 1 slice whole grain bread (page 201)
	3) 1 large orange (205)
3 oz. lean protein:	1) 3 oz. chicken (page 209)
2 fats:	1) 1 Tbsp. low-fat mayonnaise (page 210)
	2) 2 tsp. peanut butter (page 210)
Freebie:	Celery sticks (page 207)
Dinner	
4 carbohydrate choices:	1) 1/2 cups beef stew (page 204)
	2) 1/2 cups beef stew (page 204)
	3) 1/2 cups beef stew (page 204)
	4) 1 slice of Italian bread (page 201)
5 oz. lean protein:	1) 5 oz. beef in stew (page 209)
2 fats:	1) 1 tsp butter (page 211)
	2) 1 Tbsp. regular dressing (page 211)
Freebie:	Vegetable salad (page 208)

1,800 calories (with between-meal snacks)

Breakfast	**Vegetable Omelet**
3 carbohydrate choices:	1) 1 whole-grain English muffin (page 202)
	2) 1 small piece of fruit (page 204-206)
2 oz. lean protein:	1) 1 egg (1 oz.) (page 209)
	2) ¼ cup low-fat shredded cheese (pg 209)
2 fats:	1) 2 tsp. butter (page 211)
Freebies:	Veggies for the omelet (page 207-208)
Snack	
1 carbohydrate choice:	1) 8 dried apricot halves (page 206)
Lunch	**Tuna Salad Sandwich**
3 carbohydrate choices:	1) ½ wheat pita (page 201)
	2) ½ wheat pita (page 201)
	3) 1 small apple, sliced (page 204)
2 oz. lean protein:	1) 2 oz. tuna fish (page 209)
1 fat:	1) 1 Tbsp. low-fat mayonnaise (page 210)
Freebie:	Salad with 1 Tbsp. fat-free dressing (pg 208)
Snack	
1 carbohydrate choice:	1) 2 tangerines (page 205)
Dinner	**Shrimp Stir Fry**
3 carbohydrate choices:	1) 1/3 cup brown rice (page 203)
	2) 1/3 cup brown rice (page 203)
	3) 1/3 cup brown rice (page 203)
4 oz. lean protein:	1) 4 oz. shrimp (page 209)
2 fats:	1) 1 tsp olive oil (page 210)
	2) 1 tsp olive oil (page 210)
Freebies:	Stiry fry veggies (peppers and onions) pg 207
Snack	
1 carbohydrate choice:	1) 3 graham cracker squares (check the label)

Appendix B

The Portion Guide[42]

Starches

Remember that one starch choice equals fifteen grams of carbohydrate. The list below provides the serving size for one carbohydrate choice. One bread choice is usually equivalent to one ounce.

Bread

Food	**One Choice**
Bagel	¼ of a large (~4 oz.) bagel
Biscuit	1 (2 ½ -in. diameter) biscuit
Bread (most kinds: white, wheat, rye, Italian, raisin, sourdough, etc.)	1 slice (1 oz.)
Bread, low-calorie, high-fiber ("lite" bread)	2 slices
Pita	½ of a 6-in. pita
Taco shell	2 5-in. taco shells

---

[42] All tables in this section adapted from *Exchange Lists for Weight Management*, created by the American Diabetes Association and the American Dietetic Association, 2003.

Tortilla (corn, white, or wheat)	1 6-in. tortilla
English muffin	½ regular or 1 "lite" muffin
Hot dog or hamburger bun	½ bun
Pancake	1 4-in. pancake, thin
Roll, dinner	1 small (1 oz.)
Stuffing, bread	1/3 cup, prepared
Waffle	1 4-in. waffle

Cereals (all hot cereals are given in their ***prepared/cooked*** amount)

Food	**One Choice**
Bran cereal	½ cup
Cereal, hot (oatmeal, cream of wheat, grits, Kasha)	½ cup
Granola	Varies—Read Label
Puffed wheat or rice	1 ½ cups
Shredded wheat, plain	½ cup
Sugar-sweetened cereal	½ cup
Unsweetened cereals	¾ cup

Grains (all grains are given in their prepared/cooked amount)

Food	**One Choice**
Barley	1/3 cup
Bulgur	1/2 cup

Couscous	1/3 cup
Millet	1/3 cup
Pasta (all kinds, white or wheat)	1/3 cup
Quinoa (all kinds)	1/3 cup
Rice (white, brown, yellow)	1/3 cup
Tabbouleh	1/2 cup
Wild rice	1/2 cup

Starchy Vegetables (sorted by choice amount)

Food	**One Choice**
Baked beans, canned	1/3 cup
Baked potato	3 oz.
Beans (black, kidney, navy, pint, garbanzo, white, pink), canned, rinsed, cooked)	½ cup
Cassava	1/3 cup
Corn	½ cup
French fries	2 oz.
Hummus	1/3 cup
Lentils, cooked (all colors)	½ cup
Marinara (red) sauce	½ cup
Parsnips	½ cup
Peas (green, split, and black-eyed)	½ cup

Plantain	1/3 cup
Potato, mashed, or boiled	½ cup
Pumpkin, canned, no sugar added	¾ cup
Refried beans	½ cup
Succotash	½ cup
Sweet potato or yam	½ cup

Combination foods: ½ cup of a combination food is a serving and is equal to 15 grams of carbohydrate. Examples of combination foods are chili with beans, stew prepared with potatoes, rice or noodle casseroles and lasagna.

Fruit (sorted by type: fresh, canned and dried). Tip: you can weigh fresh fruit on a scale at the store to determine what size fruit you are buying.

Food	**One Choice (fresh)**
Apple	1 small (4 oz.)
Apricots	4 (5.5 oz. total)
Banana	1 small (4 oz.)
Blackberries	1 cup
Blueberries	¾ cup
Cantaloupe	1 cup cubed
Cherries	12
Figs	2 medium

Grapefruit	½ large
Grapes	17 small
Guava	2 small (2.5 oz.)
Honeydew	1 cup cubed
Mango	½ small (5.5 oz.)
Nectarine	1 medium (5.5 oz.)
Orange	1 medium (6.5 oz.)
Papaya	½ papaya
Peach	1 medium (5.5 oz.)
Pineapple	¾ cup
Plums	2 small (5 oz. total)
Raspberries	1 cup
Strawberries	1.25 cups whole berries
Tangerine	1 large or 2 small (6 oz. in total)
Watermelon	1.25 cups cubed
	One Choice (canned in light syrup)
Applesauce, unsweetened	½ cup
Apricots, canned	½ cup
Cherries, canned	½ cup
Fruit cocktail	½ cup
Kiwi	½ cup, sliced
Peaches, canned	½ cup
Pears, canned	½ cup

Pineapple, canned	½ cup
Plums, canned	½ cup
Pomegranate seeds	½ cup
	One Choice (dried)
Apples, dried	4 rings
Apricots, dried	8 halves
Dates	3 small
Dried fruits (blueberries, cherries, cranberries, mixed fruit, raisins)	2 Tbsp.
Figs	3 small
Prunes	3 prunes

Fruit Juice (sorted by choice amount)

Food	**One Choice**
Apple juice	½ cup
Cranberry juice	1/3 cup
Fruit juice, 100%, blended	1/3 cup
Grape juice	1/3 cup
Grapefruit juice	½ cup
Orange juice	½ cup
Pineapple juice	½ cup
Pomegranate juice	½ cup
Prune juice	1/3 cup

Milk (sorted by choice amount; recommended to choose 1% or skim to help with calorie intake)

Food	One Choice
Almond milk, plain	1 cup
Coconut milk, plain	1 cup
Milk, dairy, all kinds (skim, 1%, 2%, and whole; cow, goat)	1 ¼ cups
Rice milk, plain	1 cup
Soy milk, plain	1 cup
Yogurt, plain	6 oz.

Freebie Vegetables (these vegetables are considered non-starchy and can be consumed at any time in any amount)

Artichoke, artichoke hearts (in water)	Okra
Asparagus	Onions
Bean sprouts	Pea pods
Beans (green, wax, Italian)	Peppers (all kinds/colors)
Beets	Radishes
Broccoli	Rutabaga
Brussels sprouts	Sauerkraut (low-sodium)
Cabbage	Spinach
Carrots	Squash, summer (yellow and

	zucchini)
Cauliflower	Sugar snap peas
Celery	Swiss chard
Cucumber	Tomato
Eggplant	Tomato sauce (no sugar added)
Green onions or scallions	Tomato juice (low-sodium)
Greens (collard, dandelion, mustard, turnip)	Turnips
Greens, salad (arugula, endive, escarole, lettuce, radicchio, romaine)	Vegetable juice (low-sodium)
Hearts of palm (in water)	Water chestnuts
Jicama	
Kale	
Kohlrabi	
Leeks	
Mixed vegetables (broccoli, cauliflower, carrots)	
Mushrooms	

Protein (a mix of lean and medium-fat sources of protein given in 1-ounce portions; most people will get a 3- to 5-ounce portion at one or two meals a day). Choose lean proteins to help control calories since much of the fat and calories coming into your diet are usually from fatty meats and cheeses. The list below outlines primarily lean choices of protein.

Food	One Choice
Beef (95-98%), roast (chuck, round, rump, sirloin, all well-trimmed), and steak (cubed, flank, porterhouse, T-bone, tenderloin)	1 oz.
Cheese, low-fat (3 grams of fat or less per ounce)	1 oz.
Cottage or ricotta cheese; low-fat or fat-free	2 oz. (~1/4 cup)
Egg, whole	1 medium egg
Egg whites or egg substitute	2 whites or a ¼ cup egg substitute
Fish (all kinds, baked or broiled, not fried)	1 oz.
Lamb	1 oz.
Pork (ham, Canadian bacon, loin chop, roast, tenderloin)	1 oz.
Poultry (baked or broiled, without skin, fat trimmed)	1 oz.
Processed lunch meat (lean ham, turkey, roast beef)	1 oz
Shellfish of all kinds (baked or broiled, not fried)	1 oz.

Veal cutlet (baked or broiled, not breaded, not fried, loin or roast	1 oz.

Fats

Food	**One Choice**
Monounsaturated fats	
Avocado	¼ of an avocado or 1 Tbsp.
Nuts:	
Almonds	8
Cashews or mixed nuts	6
Macadamia	3
Peanuts	10
Pecans	4 halves
Pistachio	16
Nut butters (peanut, almond, cashew)	2 tsp.
Oil (olive, canola, peanut)	1 tsp.
Olives (large, black or green)	8
Polyunsaturated Fats	
Margarine, regular, all kinds	1 tsp.
Margarine, reduced-fat	1 Tbsp.
Mayonnaise, regular	1 tsp.
Mayonnaise, low-fat	1 Tbsp.
Walnuts	4 halves

Oil (corn, safflower, soybean)	1 tsp.
Salad dressing, full-fat	1 Tbsp.
Salad dressing, low-fat	2 Tbsp.
Miracle Whip® Salad Dressing, regular	2 tsp.
Miracle Whip® Salad Dressing, low-fat	1 Tbsp.
Seeds (sunflower, chia, flaxseed, pumpkin, sesame)	1 Tbsp.
Tahini (sesame) paste	2 tsp.
Saturated fats	
Bacon	1 slice
Butter, regular	1 tsp.
Butter, reduced-fat	1 Tbsp.
Butter, whipped	2 tsp.
Coconut, shredded	2 Tbsp.
Creamer (half & half or light cream)	2 Tbsp.
Cream cheese, regular	1 Tbsp.
Cream cheese, low-fat	1.5 Tbsp.
Oil (coconut, palm)	1 tsp.
Sour cream, regular	2 Tbsp.
Sour cream, low-fat	3 Tbsp.

Snacks Limit snacks to one serving of carbohydrate (a single fifteen-gram portion). You can include one ounce of lean protein if you wish, but it must be part of your total protein for the day (not in addition to your total daily protein recommendation). Ideally, a smart snack would be comprised of some kind of fruit, whole grain, or low-fat dairy. Use your portion guide to determine amounts.

Smart snacks

Carbohydrate	Protein
Fruit: Peaches or berries go great with cottage cheese!	¼ cup low-fat cottage cheese
Fruit	¼ cup low-fat ricotta cheese
Whole grain crackers (label)	1 oz. low-fat cheese (i.e. cheddar)
Whole grain crackers or rice cake (label)	1 oz. of tuna (packed in water)
Whole grain bread	1 oz. of chicken breast
Low-fat or Greek yogurt (label)	
Popcorn—3 cups popped!	

Appendix C

1,300 Calories (without snacks)

Breakfast

3 carbohydrates	1) ____________________
	2) ____________________
	3) ____________________
1 fat	1) ____________________

Lunch

3 carbohydrates	1) ____________________
	2) ____________________
	3) ____________________
2 oz. lean protein	1) ____________________
1 fat	1) ____________________
Freebies	1) ____________________

Dinner

3 carbohydrates	1) ____________________
	2) ____________________
	3) ____________________
3 oz. lean protein	1) ____________________
1 fat	1) ____________________
Freebies	1) ____________________

1,300 Calories (with between-meal snacks)

Breakfast

2 carbohydrates	1) ______________________
	2) ______________________
1 fat	1) ______________________

Snack

1 carbohydrate	1) ______________________

Lunch

2 carbohydrates	1) ______________________
	2) ______________________
2 oz. lean protein	1) ______________________
1 fat	1) ______________________
Freebies	1) ______________________

Snack

1 carbohydrate	1) ______________________

Dinner

2 carbohydrates	1) ______________________
	2) ______________________
3 oz. lean protein	1) ______________________
1 fat	1) ______________________

Snack

1 carbohydrate	1) ______________________

1,400 Calories (without snacks)

Breakfast

3 carbohydrates	1) ______________________
	2) ______________________
	3) ______________________
1 fat	1) ______________________
Freebies	1) ______________________

Lunch

3 carbohydrates	1) ______________________
	2) ______________________
	3) ______________________
3 oz. lean protein	1) ______________________
2 fats	1) ______________________
	2) ______________________
Freebies	1) ______________________

Dinner

3 carbohydrates	1) ______________________
	2) ______________________
	3) ______________________
3 oz. lean protein	1) ______________________
1 fat	1) ______________________
Freebies	1) ______________________

1,400 Calories (with between-meal snacks)

Breakfast

2 carbohydrates	1) ______________________
	2) ______________________
1 fat	1) ______________________

Snack

1 carbohydrate	1) ______________________

Lunch

2 carbohydrates	1) ______________________
	2) ______________________
3 oz. lean protein	1) ______________________
2 fats	1) ______________________
	2) ______________________
Freebies	1) ______________________

Snack

1 carbohydrate	1) ______________________

Dinner

2 carbohydrates	1) ______________________
	2) ______________________
3 oz. lean protein	1) ______________________
1 fat	1) ______________________
Freebies	1) ______________________

Snack

1 carbohydrate	1) ______________________

1,500 Calories (with evening snack)

Breakfast

3 carbohydrates	1) ________________
	2) ________________
	3) ________________
1 fat	1) ________________

Lunch

3 carbohydrates	1) ________________
	2) ________________
	3) ________________
3 oz. lean protein	1) ________________
1 fat	1) ________________
Freebies	1) ________________

Dinner

3 carbohydrates	1) ________________
	2) ________________
	3) ________________
3 oz. lean protein	1) ________________
2 fats	1) ________________
	2) ________________
Freebies	1) ________________

Snack

1 carbohydrate	1) ________________

1,500 Calories (with between-meal snacks)

Breakfast

2 carbohydrates	1) ______________________
	2) ______________________
1 fat	1) ______________________
Freebie	1) ______________________

Snack

1 carbohydrate	1) ______________________

Lunch

2 carbohydrates	1) ______________________
	2) ______________________
3 oz. lean protein	1) ______________________
1 fat	1) ______________________
Freebies	1) ______________________

Snack

1 carbohydrate	1) ______________________
Freebie	1) ______________________

Dinner

3 carbohydrates	1) ______________________
	2) ______________________
	3) ______________________
3 oz. lean protein	1) ______________________
2 fats	1) ______________________
	2) ______________________
Freebies	1) ______________________

Snack

1 carbohydrate	1) ______________________

1,600 Calories (with evening snack)

Breakfast

3 carbohydrates	1) ____________
	2) ____________
	3) ____________
1 oz. lean protein	1) ____________

Lunch

3 carbohydrates	1) ____________
	2) ____________
	3) ____________
2 oz. lean protein	1) ____________
2 fats	1) ____________
	2) ____________
Freebies	1) ____________

Dinner

4 carbohydrates	1) ____________
	2) ____________
3 oz. protein	1) ____________
2 fats	1) ____________
	2) ____________
Freebie	1) ____________

Snack

1 carbohydrate	1) ____________
1 fat	1) ____________
Freebie	1) ____________

1,600 calories (with between-meal snacks)

Breakfast

2 carbohydrates	1) ______________________
	2) ______________________
1 oz. lean protein	1) ______________________
1 fat	1) ______________________

Snack

1 carbohydrate	1) ______________________

Lunch

3 carbohydrates	1) ______________________
	2) ______________________
	3) ______________________
2 oz. lean protein	1) ______________________
1 fat	1) ______________________
Freebies	1) ______________________

Snack

1 carbohydrate	1) ______________________

Dinner

3 carbohydrates	1) ______________________
	2) ______________________
	3) ______________________
3 oz.	1) ______________________
2 fats	1) ______________________
	2) ______________________
Freebies	1) ______________________

Snack

1 carbohydrate	1) ______________________
1 fat	1) ______________________

1,700 calories (without snacks)

Breakfast

3 carbohydrates	1) ______________________
	2) ______________________
	3) ______________________
2 fats	1) ______________________
	2) ______________________
Freebie	1) ______________________

Lunch

4 carbohydrates	1) ______________________
	2) ______________________
	3) ______________________
	4) ______________________
3 oz. lean protein	1) ______________________
	2) ______________________
2 fats	1) ______________________
	2) ______________________
Freebie	1) ______________________

Dinner

4 carbohydrates	1) ______________________
	2) ______________________
	3) ______________________
	4) ______________________
5 oz. protein	1) ______________________
1 fat	1) ______________________
Freebie	1) ______________________

1,700 calories (with between-meal snacks)

Breakfast

3 carbohydrates	1) ______________________
	2) ______________________
2 oz. lean protein	1) ______________________
	2) ______________________
2 fats	1) ______________________
	2) ______________________
Freebies	1) ______________________

Lunch

3 carbohydrates	1) ______________________
	2) ______________________
2 oz. lean protein	1) ______________________
1 fat	1) ______________________
Freebie	1) ______________________

Snack

1 carbohydrate	1) ______________________

Dinner

3 carbohydrates	1) ______________________
	2) ______________________
	3) ______________________
4 oz. lean protein	1) ______________________
2 fats	1) ______________________
	2) ______________________
Freebie	1) ______________________

Snack

1 carbohydrate	1) ______________________

1,800 calories (without snacks)

Breakfast

4 carbohydrates	1) ______________________
	2) ______________________
	3) ______________________
	4) ______________________
1 fat	1) ______________________
Freebie	1) ______________________

Lunch

4 carbohydrates	1) ______________________
	2) ______________________
	3) ______________________
	4) ______________________
3 oz. lean protein	1) ______________________
2 fats	1) ______________________
	2) ______________________
Freebie	1) ______________________

Dinner

4 carbohydrates	1) ______________________
	2) ______________________
	3) ______________________
	4) ______________________
5 oz. lean protein	1) ______________________
2 fats	1) ______________________
	2) ______________________
Freebie	1) ______________________

1,800 calories (with between-meal snacks)

Breakfast

3 carbohydrates	1) ________________
	2) ________________
2 oz. lean protein	1) ________________
	2) ________________
2 fats	1) ________________
Freebies	1) ________________

Snack

1 carbohydrate	1) ________________

Lunch

3 carbohydrates	1) ________________
	2) ________________
	3) ________________
2 oz. lean protein	1) ________________
1 fat	1) ________________
Freebie	1) ________________

Snack

1 carbohydrate	1) ________________

Dinner

3 carbohydrates	1) ________________
	2) ________________
	3) ________________
4 oz. lean protein	1) ________________
2 fats	1) ________________
	2) ________________

Snack

1 carbohydrate	1) ________________

Appendix D

TIME	FOOD	AMOUNT

Appendix E[43]

Calories Burned in 60-minute activities

Moderate Physical Activity	154-pound person
Bicycling (<10 mph)	290
Dancing	330
Golf (walking and carrying clubs)	330
Hiking	370
Light gardening/yard work	330
Stretching	180
Walking (3.5 mph)	280
Weight Lifting (general light workout)	220

[43] "Calories/Hour Expended in Common Physical Activities," U.S. Department of Health and Human Services and U.S. Department of Agriculture. Dietary Guidelines for Americans, 2005. 6th Edition, Washington, DC: U.S. Government Printing Office, January 2005. https://health.gov/sites/default/files/2020-01/DGA2005.pdf#page=16.

Vigorous Physical Activity	
Aerobics	480
Bicycling (>10 mph)	590
Basketball (vigorous)	440
Heavy yard work (chopping wood) Running/jogging (5 mph)	440 590
Swimming (slow freestyle laps)	510
Walking (4.5 mph)	460
Weight lifting (vigorous effort)	440

Bibliography

American Diabetes Association. "Carb Counting and Diabetes." Accessed Jan. 15, 2015, https://www.diabetes.org/healthy-living/recipes-nutrition/understanding-carbs/carb-counting-and-diabetes.

American Diabetes Association & the American Dietetic Association. *Exchange Lists for Weight Management*, Alexandria, VA, 2003.

Bailey, Frazer, dir. *E-Motion*, 2014: Play Pictures, DVD.

Benardis, Maria. "Eating High-Vibrational Foods for Good Health and Longevity." *Huffington Post*, June 17, 2015. https://www.huffpost.com/entry/eating-high-vibrational-f_b_7596472.

Brown, Lachlan, "Karma definition: Most people are wrong about the meaning." Ideapod, May 1, 2021. https://ideapod.com/heres-great-explanation-karma-really-means-can-improve-life/.

Carlson, Andrea, and Elizabeth Frazão. *Are Healthy Foods Really More Expensive? It depends on How You Measure the Price*, EIB-96, U.S. Department of Agriculture, Economic Research Service, May 2012.

Castaldo, John E. and James F. Reed III. "The Lowering of Vascular Atherosclerotic Risk (LOVAR) Program: An Approach to Modifying Cerebral, Cardiac, and

Peripheral Vascular Disease." *Journal of Stroke and Cerebrovascular Diseases* 17, no. 1, (Winter 2008): 9-15. doi:10.1016/j.jstrokecerebrovasdis.2007.09.002.

Center for Disease Control and Prevention, "Water and Healthier Drinks." Healthy Weight, Nutrition, and Physical Activity. Last modified January 12, 2021. https://www.cdc.gov/healthywater/drinking/nutrition/index.html.

Center for Disease Control and Prevention, "Calories/Hour Expended in Common Physical Activities". Dietary Guidelines for Americans 2005. Last reviewed March 9, 2022. https://health.gov/sites/default/files/2020-01/DGA2005.pdf#page=16.

Clarity Clinic, "The Cherokee Two Wolves Story and the Power of Mindset." Oct. 16, 2020, https://www.claritychi.com/the-cherokee-two-wolves-story-and-the-power-of-mindset/.

Cleveland Clinic, "How Stress Can Make You Eat More – Or Not at All," last modified July 1, 2020, https://health.clevelandclinic.org/how-stress-can-make-you-eat-more-or-not-at-all/#:~:text=When%20you're%20feeling%20stressed,threat%20is%20causing%20the%20stress.

Dispenza, Dr. Joe. *Breaking the Habit of Being Yourself: How to Lose Your Mind and Create a New One*.

Carlsbad, CA: Hay House, Inc.,; 2012).

Escott-Stump, Sylvia. *Nutrition and Diagnosis-Related Care, Seventh Edition.* Baltimore, Maryland: Lippincott Williams & Wilkins; 2012.

Giant. "Product Search." N.d. https://giantfood.com/product-search/.

Guelinckx, Isabella, Gabriel Tavoularis, Jürgen König, Clémentine Morin, Hakam Gharbi, and Joan Gandy. "Contribution of Water from Food and Fluids to Total Water Intake: Analysis of a French and UK Population Surveys." *Nutrients* 8, no. 10, (2016): 630. doi:10.3390/nu8100630.

Haytowitz, D.B. "Effect of draining and rinsing on the sodium and water-soluble vitamin content of canned vegetables." Nutrient Data Laboratory, Beltsville Human Nutrition Research Center, Beltsville, MD. https://www.ars.usda.gov/ARSUserFiles/80400525/articles/eb11_drainedveg.pdf.

McDonald's. Menu. N.d. https://www.mcdonalds.com/us/en-us/full-menu/burgers.html.

Merriam-Webster Dictionary, s.v. "vow," accessed Feb. 24, 2021. https://www.merriam-webster.com/dictionary/vow.

MindTools, "SMART Goals," Time Management, n.d. https://www.mindtools.com/pages/article/smart-goals.htm.

Morrison, Gail, and Lisa Hark. *Medical Nutrition and Disease: A Case-Based Approach*. Cambridge, Massachusetts: Blackwell Science, 1996.

N. "How to Do Ego Work." The Holistic Psychologist, May 17, 2019,
https://theholisticpsychologist.com/how-to-do-ego-work/.

National Heart, Lung, and Blood Institute. "What causes overweight and obesity?" Last modified Dec. 1, 2016. Accessed February 18, 2021. https://www.nichd.nih.gov/health/topics/obesity/conditioninfo/cause.

National Research Council (US) Subcommittee on the Tenth Edition of the Recommended Dietary Allowances. *Recommended Dietary Allowances, 10th Edition*. (Washington, DC: National Academies Press, 1989).

"Obama After Dark: The Precious Hours Alone," *The New York Times*, July 2, 2016, https://www.nytimes.com/2016/07/03/us/politics/obama-after-dark-the-precious-hours-alone.html.

Peterson, Courtney M., Diana M. Thomas, George L. Blackburn, and Steven B. Heymsfield. "Universal equation for estimating ideal body weight and body weight at any BMI". *The American Journal of Clinical Nutrition* 103, no. 5., (2016): 1197-1203.

doi:10.3945/ajcn.115.121178.

Ramasamy, Abhilasha, François Laliberté, Shoghag A. Aktavoukian, Dominique Lejeune, Maral DerSarkissian, Cristi Cavanaugh, B. Gabriel Smolarz, Rahul Ganguly, and Mei Sheng Duh. "Direct and Indirect Cost of Obesity Among the Privately Insured in the United States." *Journal of Occupational and Environmental Medicine*: 61, no. 11, (November 2019): 877-886. doi: 10.1097/JOM.0000000000001693.

Reber, Sabrina. *Raise Your Vibration.* North Charleston, SC: CreateSpace Independent Publishing Platform; 2013.

Ryan, Donna H. and Sarah Ryan Yockey, "Weight Loss and Improvement in Comorbidity: Differences at 5%, 10%, 15%, and Over." *Current Obesity Reports* 6, no. 2, (2017): 187-194. doi:10.1007/s13679-017-0262-y.

Saltz, Gail. "Conquer your fears about losing excess weight," The Today Show, June 28, 2007, https://www.today.com/health/conquer-your-fears-about-losing-excess-weight-wbna19488269.

Shaw, George Bernard. *Everybody's Political What's What*. London: Constable and Company Ltd.; 1944.

Slavin, Joanne L. and Beate Lloyd, "Health Benefits of Fruits and Vegetables." *Advances in Nutrition* 3, no. 4, (July 2012): 506-516. doi: 10.3945/an.112.002154.

Slavin, Joanne L. and Justin Carlson, "Carbohydrates." *Advances in Nutrition* 5, no. 6, (Nov. 2014): 760-1. doi: 10.3945/an.114.006163.

Spector, Nicole. "How to train your brain to accept change, according to neuroscience," Better by Today, Nov. 12, 2018. https://www.nbcnews.com/better/health/how-train-your-brain-accept-change-according-neuroscience-ncna934011.

"The NOVA Food Classification System" in *Food, Nutrition & Fitness I: The Digestion Journey Begins with Food Choices* by EduChange (with guidance from NUPENS), Sao Paulo: 2018. https://educhange.com/wp-content/uploads/2018/09/NOVA-Classification-Reference-Sheet.pdf.

U.S. Department of Health and Human Services. *Physical Activity Guidelines for Americans, 2nd edition.* (Washington, DC: U.S. Department of Health and Human Services, 2018). https://health.gov/our-work/physical-activity/current-guidelines.

U.S. Food and Drug Administration. "Label 1." https://www.fda.gov/food/food-labeling-nutrition/nutrition-facts-label-images-download.

Wing, Rena R. and Suzanne Phelan, "Long-term weight loss maintenance." *The American Journal of Clinical Nutrition* 82, no. 1, (2005): 222S-225S.

https://doi.org/10.1093/ajcn/82.1.222S.

World Health Organization. "Healthy Diet." Apr. 29, 2020, https://www.who.int/news-room/fact-sheets/detail/healthy-diet.

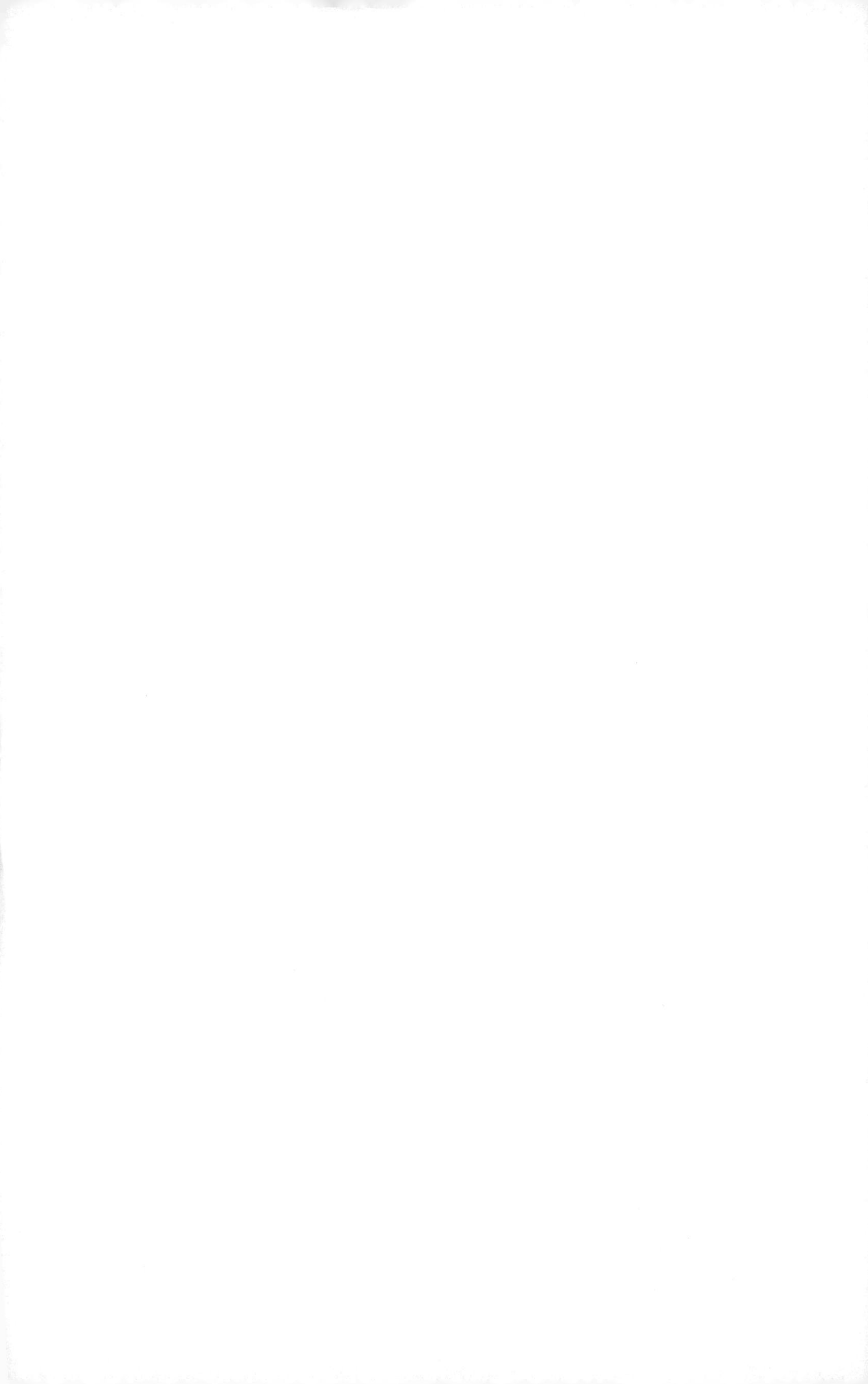

www.ingramcontent.com/pod-product-compliance
Ingram Content Group UK Ltd.
Pitfield, Milton Keynes, MK11 3LW, UK
UKHW021905190726
13853UKWH00002B/522

9 798894 200972